patrick
HOLFORD

SAY NO TO
HEART
DISEASE

piatkus

PIATKUS

First published in Great Britain in 1998 by Piatkus Books
This updated and expanded edition first published 2012 by Piatkus

Typeset in Berkeley by Phoenix Photosetting, Chatham, Kent
Printed and bound in Great Britain by CPI (UK) Ltd, Croydon, CR0 4YY

Papers used by Piatkus are from well-managed forests
and other responsible sources.

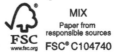

MIX
Paper from
responsible sources
FSC® C104740

Piatkus
An imprint of
Little, Brown Book Group
Carmelite House
50 Victoria Embankment
London EC4Y 0DZ

An Hachette UK Company
www.hachette.co.uk

www.piatkus.co.uk

Contents

Acknowledgements

I am immensely grateful to Nina Omotoso, my nutritional therapist researcher, and also to Jerome Burne, Dr Stephen Sinatra,
Dr Fedon Lindberg and many other switched-on doctors and
researchers who have helped to keep me up to date with the ocean of
studies on nutrition, medicine and heart disease. I am also grateful to
the 'hands-on' feedback from the participants in our Zest4Life groups
who have shared their experiences of trying out the principles in this
book. Also, a big thanks to the editorial team at Little, Brown – Gill
Bailey, Jillian Stewart and Jan Cutler – and everyone else who has
helped to get this information out to as many people as possible.
Most of all I am grateful to my wife, Gaby, who is always there for me.

Guide to Abbreviations, Measures and References

Conversions

European and American laboratories use different measures to record test results. Figures in this book are in mmol/l and pmol/l, the UK measures (although blood cholesterol and triglyceride levels are given in UK and US measurements in the charts). If necessary, your results can be easily converted using the following rules.

To convert **blood glucose** readings:
Multiply the mg/dL (US) by 0.0555 to get mmol/l (UK).

To convert **glycosylated haemoglobin (glycated haemoglobin A1, A1C, HbAIC)** readings:
Multiply 'proportion of total haemoglobin' by 100 to get 'per cent of total haemoglobin'.

To convert **insulin** readings:
Multiply the μIU/mL (US) by 0.6.945 to get mmol/l (UK).

To convert **total cholesterol**, HDL and LDL readings:
Multiply the mg/dl (US) by 0.0259 to get mmol/l (UK).

To convert **triglyceride** readings:
Multiply the mg/dl (US) by 0.0113 to get mmol/l (UK).

Vitamins

1 gram (g) = 1,000 milligrams (mg) = 1,000,000 micrograms (mcg, also written as µg)

1mcg of retinol (1mcg RE) = 3.3ius of vitamin A

1mcg RE of beta-carotene = 6mcg of beta-carotene

100iu of vitamin D = 2.5mcg

100iu of vitamin E = 67mg

Most vitamins are measured in milligrams or micrograms. Vitamins A, D and E used to be measured in International Units (iu), a measurement designed to standardise the various forms of these vitamins, which have different potencies.

1 pound (lb) = 16 ounces (oz)/450g

2lb 4oz = 1 kilogram (kg)

1 pint = 600ml/20fl oz

1¾ pints = 1 litre

In this book 'calories' means kilocalories (kcals)

References and Further Sources of Information

In each part of the book, you'll find numbered references. These refer to research papers listed in the References section on page 279, and are there for readers who want to study this subject in depth. More details on most of these studies can be found on the Internet, at PubMed, a service of the US National Library of Medicine. This is where you can access most of the studies mentioned (see http://www.ncbi.nlm.nih.gov/pubmed/).

On page 300 you will find a list of the best books to read to enable you to dig deeper into the topics covered. You will also find many of the topics touched on in this book covered in detail in feature articles available at www.patrickholford.com. If you want to stay up to date with all that is new and exciting in this field, we recommend you subscribe to Patrick Holford's 100% Health newsletter, details of which are on the website.

CAUTION

Although all the nutrients and dietary changes referred to in this book have been proven safe, those seeking help for specific medical conditions are advised to consult a qualified nutritional therapist, clinical nutritionist, nutritionally oriented doctor or equivalent health professional. The recommendations given in this book are solely intended as education and information, and should not be taken as medical advice. Neither the author nor the publisher accepts liability for readers who choose to self-prescribe.

If you are on medication for a heart condition, consult your doctor before adjusting any medication. If you are on medication for diabetes, it is especially important to monitor your blood sugar levels and to consult your doctor if you wish to adjust your medication. Do not change your medication without consulting your doctor.

All supplements should be kept out of the reach of infants and children.

Introduction

When I wrote the first edition of this book, in 1998, many of the key drivers of heart disease that I proposed – high blood sugar levels, lack of omega-3 fats and magnesium, high homocysteine and lipoprotein(a) – were largely unknown in mainstream medicine. Now, 14 years on, the small hill of evidence backing up an optimum-nutrition approach to heart disease has turned into a large mountain, yet, with a few exceptions such as the more widespread prescription of omega-3, very few people with cardiovascular risk are being given the right advice about what to eat and supplement.

Too many people are told to eat a low-fat, low-cholesterol diet despite clear evidence that this doesn't work; too few are given vitamin B_3 (niacin) to lower cholesterol despite the fact that it is safer, and it lowers cholesterol better, than statin drugs, nor are they given vitamin C, now well established to substantially reduce risk, and almost none are given magnesium, an inexpensive mineral that lowers blood pressure, reduces heart attack and stroke risk, and maximises recovery.

Back in the 1990s, one in five men and one in nine women were dying of heart disease before they reached the age of 75. I had hoped, and naively expected, that this trend would be reversed by applying the science of optimum nutrition to cardiovascular medicine. After all, it is cheap, safe and effective. But, in some respects, the situation has become worse not better, especially for women. It used to be the case that many more men than women died from heart disease, but in recent years the numbers have evened out, with more women than men dying from strokes in particular. Advances in medicine mean that more people survive a stroke or heart attack, but how is their quality of life affected? If you have had such an event, it can be a wake-up call: a chance to examine what caused the problem and to reverse that risk. If you haven't had a stroke or heart attack, one ounce of prevention is worth several pounds of cure.

Heart disease is the number-one cause of premature death

More people die prematurely from diseases of the heart and arteries than from anything else – 150,000 a year in England alone – roughly half from heart attacks and a quarter from strokes.[1] (A stroke occurs when the flow of blood to the brain is disrupted, resulting in a sudden disabling attack or loss of consciousness.) At least 20,000 deaths occur prematurely in people under the age of 75. In the UK, there are an estimated 2.6 million people living with the condition, and angina (the most common symptom of coronary heart disease) affects 2 million people. Worldwide, over 8 million women die every year from heart disease. In America alone there are about 8 million women living with heart disease.

There is nothing natural about dying from heart disease. Many cultures in the world do not experience a particularly high incidence of strokes or heart attacks. British people, for example, have nine times as much heart disease by middle age as the Japanese. If you are a woman and you live in Scotland, your chances of having a heart attack are eight times higher than if you live in Spain.[2] Why?

Autopsies performed on Egyptian mummies of people who died in 3000 BC show signs of deposits in the arteries but no actual blockages that would have resulted in a stroke or heart attack. Despite how obvious the signs of hearts attacks are (severe chest pain, cold sweats, nausea, a fall in blood pressure and a weak pulse), in the 1930s they were so rare that it took a specialist to make the diagnosis. According to American health records, the incidence per 100,000 people of heart attack was zero in 1890. By 1970 it had risen to 340. Although deaths did occur from other forms of heart disease, including calcified valves, rheumatic heart and other congenital defects, the incidence of actual blockages in the arteries, which cause strokes or heart attacks, was minimal. Heart disease used to be rare in India and Africa but is now endemic, especially in regions that have a more 'Westernised' diet and lifestyle. Why? I will be exploring the reasons for these differences in detail, but first, in Part 1, I will be bringing you up to speed with the dynamics of heart disease and explaining what a diagnosis actually means, as well as the risk factors such as blood pressure and blood fats.

Twenty years less of life

The cost of heart disease is, on average, 20 years less life. For those who survive a massive heart attack or stroke it may mean decades of compromised living. Yet heart attacks, heart failure and strokes are largely preventable diseases with highly familiar risk factors, such as poor nutrition, smoking, excess alcohol, obesity and lack of exercise. Investing a bit of time and energy in finding out what's going to make all the difference to you can literally add years to your life as well as life to your years.

If you've just been diagnosed with some form of heart disease – angina, hypertension (high blood pressure), thrombosis, a stroke or heart attack – your doctor is probably unlikely to focus on these risk factors, although you may be given some general advice to lose weight, exercise and eat a 'well-balanced diet'. Instead, you'll probably be prescribed a cocktail of drugs to lower your cholesterol, bring down your blood pressure and thin your blood. The trouble is these medications all interfere with some aspect of your body's chemistry and none are necessary long term if you address the underlying causes of heart disease (in this book I will call the family of blood-vessel related diseases – strokes, heart attacks, angina, high blood pressure – heart disease).

The combined strategy of changing your diet, improving your lifestyle, and taking the right supplements is likely to be far more effective than taking prescribed drugs for both preventing and reversing cardiovascular disease, without the side effects. If you are on medication and take these steps to reduce your risk, and thereby achieve normalisation of the signs in your body that show that you are developing cardiovascular disease (known as biochemical markers), there should be no need to continue taking cardiovascular medication unless you have suffered physical, irreversible damage. Long-term medication is often only necessary if you are unwilling to make the necessary changes to your diet and lifestyle; however, do not change any prescribed medication without first consulting your doctor and re-evaluating the measurable risk factors that medication targets.

You can normalise your blood pressure without drugs

David is an example of how lifestyle changes can have dramatic effects:

Case Study: David

David had suffered from high blood pressure for years and was on long-term medication, but when he started following my Heart-friendly Diet (a healthy 'low-GL diet' based on choosing carbohydrates that slowly release in the body) the combination of the diet and drugs was too much and his blood pressure went from too high to too low. He had to stop the drugs to achieve a healthy, normal blood pressure. In his own words:

> 'Two months later I had to see the cardiology professor again and I took along my own blood pressure figures for him to analyse. He was astonished and highly delighted with such brilliant figures from me. Then I broke the news to him, that those figures had been achieved without any medication at all! The initial look of

horror on his face changed to total fascination when I explained that all I had done was follow your low-GL diet.

'He carried out more tests on me, including a potassium-to-salt ratio, which showed that my salt levels were so low that he said I was just like someone from a particular tribe in Africa that does not suffer from any blood pressure problems whatsoever. By contrast, he said that my potassium levels were so high that he thought I must be eating fruit and vegetables all day long in order to achieve this. I said no, I just follow the low-GL diet. In fact, prior to the diet I was constantly eating fruit during the day but without any benefit to my blood pressure. Another benefit of the low-GL diet was that my cholesterol dropped from 5.7 to 4.6. I have now been on the diet for three years and have not had to revert to blood pressure tablets.'

The ten keys to staying free from heart disease for life

Eating a low-GL diet is one of ten key factors for keeping healthy and keeping your blood pressure down. There are other keys, such as getting enough magnesium and omega-3 fats, or taking co-enzyme Q_{10} (CoQ$_{10}$) and carnitine if you have heart problems. In Part 2 you'll learn about the ten key factors that ensure you keep heart-healthy throughout your life. There is simply no need to suffer from heart disease at any age.

These keys include:

- Achieving perfect cholesterol without drugs.

- Eating the right kind of fats to halve your risk of a heart attack.

- Becoming a master of your blood sugar control, thereby preventing arterial damage.

- Following simple, five-minute techniques that teach you how to undo stress.

- Learning what you can and can't drink to reduce your risk.

- Lowering your homocysteine, an independent risk factor that is more important than your cholesterol level.

- Lowering lipoprotein(a), another key risk factor that probably hasn't been checked by your health professional.

- Getting the most antioxidant protection to keep your blood vessels young and flexible.

- Understanding how to get your mineral balance right and the importance of magnesium for perfect blood pressure.

- Learning how to switch off your heart-disease-promoting genes and how to switch on the heart-protective genes.

Put all these factors together and you have a potent package for saying no to heart disease for your whole life. The experiences of my first teacher, Dr Carl Pfeiffer, confirm this. (I first met Dr Pfeiffer in the 1970s when he introduced me to the power of nutritional therapy for mental illness when I was studying as a psychologist.)

Dr Pfeiffer had a massive heart attack at the age of 51 and was told that he would not survive without a pacemaker and medication, and even then for no more than ten years. He chose neither and instead examined the true underlying causes, which led him to radically change his diet and start taking supplements. He lived to be 80 years old, seeing patients six days a week, and was active to the last minute. My other teachers, Drs Linus Pauling, Abram Hoffer and Roger Williams, all lived well into their nineties without any form of heart disease, never retiring or losing their razor-sharp minds.

With regard to myself, at the age of 54 at the time of writing, my vital statistics – cholesterol, blood pressure and pulse – remain exactly the same as they were when I was in my twenties. My homocysteine level, a key risk factor, is at the same average level as a teenager's. I can still climb mountains with my super-fit daughter despite a daily maintenance exercise routine of only 15 minutes (although you would need more than this to recover from a heart problem).

Working with your doctor
to reduce medication

Obviously, if you've had a heart attack or have very high blood pressure, I am not suggesting that you throw your drugs away. Let your doctor know that you want to pursue nutritional and lifestyle changes to minimise your need for medication.

Part 3 gives you concrete strategies for lowering cholesterol and blood pressure, as well as maximising your recovery if you've had a heart attack or stroke so that you can get started on the road to improved health right away.

It's a good idea to establish the goal that would make it no longer necessary for you to have medication; for example, a cholesterol measure below 5, or blood pressure below 130/85. Then, as you start to incorporate the nutritional changes I recommend, you can monitor the effect. Some drugs become dangerous to take when you've achieved the goal; for example, when normalising your blood pressure or cholesterol, too low a cholesterol level is as bad as one that is too high.

If you're on blood-thinning drugs such as aspirin or warfarin, speak to your doctor before taking concentrated supplements of omega-3 fish oils, gingko biloba or vitamin E above 300mg, because your medical practice may want to monitor your INR and platelet-adhesion index and consider reducing the drug accordingly. If you can achieve perfect blood without drugs this has to be the better way. The same is true with cholesterol and blood pressure.

As your vital heart statistics improve, any doctor worth their salt will want to reduce your medication accordingly, because almost all drugs have undesirable side effects. There's no point in taking medication if you don't need it; however, many drugs are given out far too freely to people for whom they are likely to be of no benefit at all. This includes the cholesterol-lowering statins given to women as a preventative, and a daily aspirin. The evidence shows that these simply do not work, yet they have achieved almost cult status in basic medical advice. I'll be exploring the best and the worst drugs in Chapter 6 and will let you know which nutrients could interfere with the action of a drug (very few) and, more importantly, which drugs interfere with the action of a nutrient, making you even more deficient.

Unfortunately, too many doctors and dieticians, out of fear and ignorance, may tell you there's no evidence that you can make these changes through nutritional and lifestyle changes and they'd rather you didn't take supplements in case they interfere with your medication. I had first-hand experience of this recently when a dear friend, in his seventies, had just come out of a coma and was in the hospital's stroke recovery unit. I presented a paper, with all the references of all the nutrients, proven to be safe, that could help recovery, and the tests that should be run – including homocysteine and his vitamin D status (he had had three months with no direct sunlight and his vitamin D status was in all probability very low). Despite the fact that there could only be benefit from testing and adding in any deficient nutrients, they refused to run the tests or give the supplements, instead giving him an RDA (Recommended Daily Allowance) multivitamin in recognition that a hospital diet may not provide enough nutrients, plus one of the least effective blood pressure drugs with the most side effects. As many studies have proven, however, RDA levels of nutrients just aren't enough to make a difference, and especially when your body is out of balance, because you need a much higher intake of nutrients to restore your body to good health.

If you encounter this kind of closed-mind resistance, it is best to find a medical team who will support you, not hinder you, in taking responsibility for your own health, and perhaps work with a registered nutritional therapist who can help present the evidence for adding a nutrition-based strategy to your prevention or recovery programme. Be wary of any advice that you have to take medication 'for life'. In my experience, this is rarely necessary if you truly follow an optimum nutrition programme.

Your Healthy-heart Action Plan

Whether you are reading this book for prevention, to help you or someone you know recover from cardiovascular disease, a heart attack or a stroke, or to make sure the tell-tale signs you've started to develop don't go any further, and will hopefully recede, you will be pleasantly surprised, and perhaps amazed, to find how much evidence there already is that optimum nutrition really can help you to say no to heart disease. The trouble is that doctors simply aren't taught this in medical school, and since nutrients are not patentable, hence not significantly profitable, there's no industry pushing postgraduate education. The mainstay of modern medicine is still based on the prescribing of drugs and it is hard for a doctor to step out of the box. In the UK, doctors are remunerated for testing, and lowering, cholesterol and often give cholesterol-lowering drugs that don't actually reduce heart disease risk. Few doctors have the experience, or the confidence, to tackle heart disease with a largely nutrition-based strategy. That means it is up to you to find out what you can do for yourself.

In Part 4 you'll discover how to build your own Healthy-heart Action Plan depending on your current level of health, together with the practical information you will need on my Heart-friendly Diet, supplements, exercise and stress reduction. If you wish, you can consult a registered nutritional therapist to help devise a plan of action for you (see Resources) who will use these tried-and-tested principles to deliver measurable results in weeks, not months, giving you the confidence to keep going and change the baseline of what you eat and how you live. But you can also get these results by working through the book.

Back in the 4th century BC Hippocrates, the father of modern medicine, said 'what's good for the heart is good for the mind'. You'll be pleased to discover that there are good side effects to the optimum-nutrition approach to heart disease, such as more energy, a sharper mind, a more balanced mood and less pain. It's a win–win situation all round and it's yours for the taking.

Wishing you the best of health,
Patrick Holford

PART 1

THE DYNAMICS OF HEART DISEASE

One in two men and women die from heart disease. More people die prematurely, and many more suffer, from diseases of the heart and arteries than from anything else. Decades of research have made it clear that there is not one single cure. It's more complicated than that. This Part explains the dynamics of cardiovascular health, how your heart and arteries work, what the critical risk factors are and what measurements, such as your blood pressure, cholesterol and blood-fat levels, actually mean. You'll also learn why you may be offered certain drugs, what they do and how effective they are.

CHAPTER 1

Your Healthy Heart Check: Identify Your Critical Risk Factors

No disorder has been more thoroughly investigated than heart disease. Now the fruits of all this research are yours to benefit from. Strangely though, all the pieces of information have yet to be compiled and presented as a clear strategy for eliminating the risk of heart disease. That is the purpose of this book, and you may be amazed to find that you can reduce your risk almost completely.

You can divide your critical risk factors into things that you do or have, such as your diet, smoking or excess weight, and measurements of something going on in your body, such as your cholesterol or homocysteine levels. The usual assumption is that lowering a measure that is associated with a higher risk, such as your cholesterol or homocysteine, will always reduce your risk. Although this is usually true, it isn't always the case.

Also, we tend to be sold a very linear story, such as 'cholesterol blocks the arteries, therefore eat less cholesterol by avoiding, for example, eggs, and take drugs that lower cholesterol'. In this particular case, having a high cholesterol level is a predictive marker of heart disease, but it isn't caused by high dietary intake. Avoiding eggs won't make any difference, as you'll discover later. One of the main reasons cholesterol goes up is eating too much sugar and refined carbohydrates, as well as having too much stress. Both too much sugar and concomitantly high insulin (the result of a diet high in sugar and refined carbohydrates) damages the arteries and raises blood pressure. Simply taking a drug that stops you making cholesterol has little effect if you don't change your diet.

Why lowering cholesterol isn't the full story

In the case of cholesterol, it's not a particularly good predictive marker. The odds are that if you have a heart attack you don't also have high cholesterol. A massive US survey of 136,905 patients found that the majority of those hospitalised for a heart attack had normal cholesterol levels.[1] Although you don't want to have a high cholesterol level it also means that you shouldn't think you are in the clear just because your cholesterol level is normal. It is only one of a number of risk factors, and not the most predictive at that.

The trouble is that, due to extensive marketing of cholesterol-lowering drugs, doctors have become too focused on this and are, at least in the UK, financially rewarded if they test your cholesterol, and then again if they lower your level, which is easiest to do by giving you a cholesterol-lowering drug. It is not the drug that most reduces your risk, however, but changing your diet and lifestyle, which although it requires more effort is much more effective.

Among elderly people, for example, cholesterol is a very poor predictor of cardiovascular-disease death, as is a widely used index of conventional risk factors called the Framingham Risk Score, based on assessments of blood pressure, cholesterol, ECG (electrocardiograph), diabetes and smoking. The best predictor by far is your homocysteine level, according to a study published in the *British Medical Journal*.[2] (Homocysteine is a critical risk factor that I'll be exploring in detail.) The study found that if a person's homocysteine level was above 13, which is not much higher than the average for a 50-year-old, it predicted no less than two-thirds of all deaths five years on.

You can lower it easily by simply taking homocysteine-lowering B vitamins. According to some studies, if you've already had a heart attack, lowering homocysteine doesn't appear to lower the risk of another heart attack, but it does lower the risk of stroke. (Although, as you will see later, this lack of benefit may be more to do with common heart-disease drugs interfering with the ability of B vitamins to work.) Homocysteine-lowering B vitamins are more effective in reducing your risk if your homocysteine level is high to start with, as you'd expect. Less promising results with B vitamins in those with heart disease and on medication do not alter the fact that homocysteine is an excellent predictor of cardiovascular risk, better than cholesterol, yet in the UK few doctors ever check it. In Germany doctors routinely check homocysteine, running millions of tests a year. Other risk factors include your level of blood fats (triglycerides), your blood sugar balance (reflected by your HbA1c level) and something called lipoprotein(a).

Why the bigger picture is so important

It is very important to look at all risk factors, and the predictive markers, and to do your best to reduce them all. Don't put all your eggs in one basket, such as concentrating on your cholesterol level.

The chart on page 6 shows the major known risk factors for heart disease, and the percentage decreased risk you can expect by going from a bad score or diet to an optimum score, diet and lifestyle. The good news is that every one, except a genetic predisposition, can be eliminated by relatively simple, painless dietary and lifestyle changes.

What are the risk factors?

Look at the list of risk factors on page 6. All can be corrected by making simple dietary and lifestyle changes, and by doing so you may reduce your risk by the estimated percentages:

Medical statistics

High blood fats (triglycerides)	70 per cent*
High glycosylated haemoglobin (HbA1c)	68 per cent
High blood cholesterol (low HDL, high LDL)	60 per cent
High blood homocysteine	50 per cent
High lipoprotein(a)	50 per cent
High blood pressure	30 per cent
Insulin resistance	30 per cent
C-reactive protein (CRP)	20 per cent

Diet

A high-GL (glycemic load) diet** (especially in women)	50 per cent
Too much meat and dairy products	50 per cent
Too much alcohol	50 per cent
Too little antioxidant-rich foods and nutrients	50 per cent
Too little B vitamins	50 per cent
Too little potassium, magnesium and calcium	50 per cent
Too little omega-3 fats (from fish and seeds)	40 per cent
Too little fresh fruit and vegetables	30 per cent
Too much salt (sodium)	25 per cent
Too little vitamin D	20 per cent
Too much dietary saturated fat	20 per cent

Lifestyle

Smoking (20 cigarettes a day)	70 per cent
Lack of aerobic and resistance exercise	50 per cent
Too much stress	50 per cent
Overweight	30 per cent
Lack of sunlight (vitamin D)	10 per cent

Genetic predisposition	5 per cent

*All of these percentages are very approximate, based on current research and will be explored in detail in the following chapters. A good, but slightly old review of research and risk factors is 'Nutritional Aspects of Cardiovascular Disease', Department of Health, 1994.

**A high-GL (glycemic load) diet is one that is high in refined cereals and sugars.

Please note, however, that you can't take these percentage reductions too literally. And you can't just add all the percentages together, because many of these factors overlap, but the point is that we already do know how to effectively eliminate the vast majority of risks for heart disease. To illustrate this let's say you are an average person with an average diet and lifestyle, with an average 50 per cent risk of dying from heart disease. Now you decide to eat more fruit and vegetables (which are rich in antioxidant vitamins, potassium, magnesium and calcium), you follow a low-GL diet (one that is low in fast-releasing carbohydrates such as sugar and refined foods) and you stop adding salt to your food. This will lower your blood pressure, reducing your risk by 25 per cent.

If you then stop smoking 20 cigarettes a day, you reduce your risk by another 50 per cent. If you decide to supplement vitamin C and B complex to your diet, the vitamin C will lower your cholesterol and homocysteine, thereby reducing your risk by 50 per cent; the B complex will also lower your homocysteine (which is a toxin for the arteries), further reducing your risk. If you also supplement vitamin D and spend more time outdoors, that reduces your risk by 20 per cent. Then, if you cut your alcohol consumption down, but not out (because some alcohol is protective), to, on average, one drink a day, you will further reduce your risk by 50 per cent. If you start exercising three times a week, that's another 50 per cent risk reduction. Exercise also helps to bring down your stress level, but you can also learn some simple techniques such as HeartMath (explained in detail later) to keep your stress levels under control. Start eating more fish, such as salmon and tuna (providing essential omega-3 fats), and less meat and you have an associated 40 per cent reduction in risk.

Could you reduce your risk completely?

Even if these are over-exaggerations of the kinds of risk reduction you can achieve, just how far do you need to go before you have no risk at all?

7

In truth, it is not exactly known, because studies haven't been done on the combined effects of all these well-proven preventions. The chances of virtually eliminating all risk are, however, very high indeed, even if you are genetically predisposed to heart disease.

One study that tried to evaluate the significant contributors to overall risk of having a heart attack was the INTERHEART study, involving people from all over the world to get a truly global picture.[3] Their conclusion was that 'Abnormal lipids [e.g. cholesterol, triglycerides, etc.], smoking, hypertension, diabetes, abdominal obesity, psychosocial factors, consumption of fruits, vegetables, and alcohol, and regular physical activity account for most of the risk of myocardial infarction worldwide in both sexes and at all ages in all regions.' By 'most' they meant a 90 per cent reduction, and they recommended that prevention strategies should focus on these key drivers.

Another important point to make is that what you need to do to prevent heart disease is much less than what you need to do to reverse it. You need much larger amounts of nutrients, for example, to lower a high homocysteine level, or to restore blood sugar balance, than you need to maintain it in a healthy range. I'll explain what you need for both scenarios in Parts 2 and 3.

Vital statistics you should aim to improve

The main measures that indicate you have risk or have reduced risk that should be measured in any thorough medical screening are your blood pressure, cholesterol levels (your HDL to LDL ratio and your total cholesterol level), triglyceride levels, glycosylated haemoglobin (HbA1c – a measure of your ability to keep your blood sugar level in balance) and your homocysteine level. Let's look at each one separately.

Your blood pressure This is measured as, for example, 120/76 mmHg. The top figure is the systolic blood pressure, the bottom figure the diastolic blood pressure. It's the bottom figure – your diastolic blood pressure – that's the most important. If your blood pressure is above

140/90, you have a much greater risk of heart disease. In fact, roughly every 10-point increase above 76 (your diastolic pressure) doubles your risk of death from cardiovascular disease. I explain how this works in Chapter 2.

Your triglyceride level This reflects the level of fats in your bloodstream and is raised by eating diets that are high in fat and sugar, or by excessive alcohol. It's a very good, and often neglected, predictor of heart disease risk. Your triglyceride level should be below 1.7 mmol/l although the optimal is below 1mmol/l. As a rough indicator, every 0.5mmol/l potentially doubles your risk. If it is high, go on a low-GL diet as explained in this book. You don't have to be on a low-fat diet, just have more omega-3 fats from fish, raw nuts and seeds, and less fatty meat, dairy products and junk food. Chapter 3 explains why it's not really just about eating less fat.

Your homocysteine level This is measured in micromoles per litre (mcmol/l); for example, as 7mcmol/l. A healthy score is below 7. As a rough indicator, with every 5-point increase above 7mcmol/l you double your risk of death from cardiovascular disease. You certainly don't want to have a level above 10mcmol/l. Above 15mcmol/l and you have probably quadrupled your risk. This test is available as a home test kit if your doctor won't measure it for you. The solution is a change in both diet and lifestyle, plus B vitamins, as I explain in Chapter 10.

Your glycosylated haemoglobin level This is also called HbA1c and measures the percentage of red blood cells that are effectively sugar-coated, giving you an average figure of how many blood sugar spikes you have, which cause damage to your arteries. You usually get a score of between 4 and 9 per cent. Below 5 per cent is very healthy. Above 7 per cent and you are likely to be diabetic, or likely to become diabetic. If you have a level of 6.5 per cent you've probably doubled your risk of heart disease compared to if it had been just 0.5 per cent lower; however, standard blood tests might measure your fasting glucose first, which should be low. The solution is to eat a low-GL diet, as well as supplementing chromium, as I explain in Chapter 8.

This test is available as a home test kit if your doctor won't measure it for you.

Your cholesterol level This is broken down into your total cholesterol, your LDL ('bad') cholesterol and your HDL ('good') cholesterol. You should have a low LDL cholesterol (ideally below 2.6mmol/l), a high HDL cholesterol (ideally above 1.6mmol/l), and a total cholesterol of not less than 3.9mmol/l and not more than 5.2mmol/l. As a rough indicator, with every 1-point increase in your total cholesterol above 5, you double your risk of death from cardiovascular disease. With every 1-point increase in LDL, you double your risk, and with every 0.5 decrease in HDL below 1.5mmol/l, you double your risk. So you should have a high HDL and low cholesterol. The ratio of cholesterol to HDL is particularly predictive. According to one study it accounts for 37 per cent of one's overall risk of heart disease.[4]

Even better is the ratio between triglycerides and HDL. This should be as low as possible. Chapters 4 and 7 give you the low-down on cholesterol.

There are other important measures, such as your platelet adhesion index, fibrinogen and lipoprotein(a) levels, which all affect the stickiness of your blood and the preponderance to atherosclerosis (hardening of the arteries); lipoprotein(a); and C-reactive protein level, which indicates inflammation in the arteries – all these will be discussed later in the book. It's essential that your doctor measures all of these important risk factors as well. I'll explain why they are important to know for a full-scale personalised prevention policy and recovery plan.

Are you suffering from metabolic syndrome?

A number of the above risk indicators are grouped together to diagnose a condition called metabolic syndrome. This describes a common pattern of shift in your body's biology that not only increases the risk of heart disease but also of diabetes, cancer and many other conditions. Reversing metabolic syndrome is one of the essential keys to preventing and reversing heart disease.

Einstein apparently once said, 'Not everything that counts can be counted and not everything that can be counted counts.' Modern medicine loves quantifiable factors such as these indicators. Often your apparent state of health is determined by a drop in one of these scores, and drugs are sold with the intention of changing these scores. As we explore these in more detail in this book bear in mind that something can be a predictive marker of risk, but not necessarily part of the cause. One doesn't necessarily lead to the other. Sometimes a treatment might, for example, lower cholesterol but not stop heart attack deaths. This is the kind of thing we have to examine.

Other risk factors

There are other factors of tremendous importance but which are not easily measured, such as your stress level, how much exercise you take and your overall diet. Since these cannot be easily quantified by medical professionals they are usually assigned to general platitudes about the need to exercise more, eat well and try to reduce stress. But all these things are much harder to do than to take a pill, even though the likelihood is that it was not attending to these things that got you to where you are today.

Is heart disease acquired or inherited?

One often asked question is to what extent one's risk is genetic. Some people are told they have genetically high cholesterol, or triglycerides, or some other risk factor. Cardiovascular disease often runs in families – a factor which led to the debate on whether we inherit it from our parents or acquire it through diet and lifestyle habits. The answer is both. As you'll discover, your level of cholesterol, triglycerides, homocysteine and lipoprotein(a) all predict an increased risk of cardiovascular disease. The tendency to overproduce these appears to be, in part, inherited, yet your diet can prevent these risk factors ever emerging and can also reverse the risk once developed. This means that even if you have a family history of cardiovascular disease you don't have to suffer. In any case, family histories of disease often have nothing to do with inheriting genetic predispositions as such, rather they occur from inheriting certain lifestyle and dietary habits that put you at risk. In both cases the good news is that you can do something about it. This is especially encouraging, since it is a lot easier to improve your diet than to change your genes. And the earlier you start the better.

Does heart disease start in the womb?

Thanks to the extraordinary work of Professor Barker and colleagues at the Environmental Epidemiology Unit at Southampton University we now know that cardiovascular disease can be 'programmed' during foetal development, depending on the nutrition a foetus receives from its mother during pregnancy.

The researchers found that those born with a low birth weight had a high risk of hypertension, diabetes and cardiovascular disease later in life. Other surveys had found double the risk of cardiovascular disease or diabetes in infants who were thin at birth or short in terms of body length.

To investigate this new risk factor more fully, Professor Barker collaborated with researchers from Helsinki University Central Hospital in Finland in a remarkable study of 3,302 men born in the hospital between the years of 1924 and 1933.[5] Since Finland has among the highest cardiovascular disease rates in the world, and an excellent system for recording details at birth, here was a unique opportunity to put the 'foetal programming' theory to the test. They tracked down each of these 3,302 men to determine whether they were alive, and, if so, their health, and, if not, their cause of death. What they found confirmed the strong connection between foetal development and a later risk of cardiovascular disease and also gave strong clues as to why.

The men with the highest rates of death from cardiovascular disease were those who were thin at birth, where the placenta was low in weight, and where the mother was short and fat. Professor Barker explains this finding in the following way. If a mother is grossly undernourished during foetal development and infancy she will grow up to be shorter. As her nutrition improves in adulthood she gains weight, but not height, so ends up short and fat. The ability to produce a large, healthy placenta, which is the network of blood vessels that nourish her offspring during pregnancy, is more dependent on her own early development not just her level of nutrition during pregnancy. So her offspring will not have as good a supply of nutrients during the development of her foetus, despite her own improved nutrition. As a consequence her baby is more likely to be short and thin, indicating poor foetal nutrition, and will have a greater risk of diabetes and cardiovascular disease later in life. Conversely, a taller well-nourished mother giving birth to a chubby baby means minimal risk of cardiovascular disease later in life.

Survival of the fattest

But what exactly is going on in the womb that programmes disease decades later? The theory is that the developing foetus adapts to the inadequate nutrition by changing its metabolism and organ structure, favouring protection of the developing brain. The end result is that the infant is effectively born with insulin resistance (problems with blood sugar control: the hormone insulin becomes less able to lower sugar in the blood, potentially leading to diabetes later in life). This altered metabolism of glucose and resistance to insulin programmes the infant to develop blood sugar and cardiovascular problems later in life.

Of course, if you happen to have been born small and thin to a mother who was short and fat this news may not be exactly welcome; however, what we now know about insulin resistance is that a specific nutrition strategy, including the right balance of protein

13

and carbohydrate, plus key amino acids, vitamins and minerals, may be able to reprogramme metabolism to reduce the risk. Also, knowing this, early nutritional intervention in infants born short and thin in relation to their gestational age may have a significant effect in reducing the risk of cardiovascular disease later in life.

The first 1,000 days

It isn't just what happens during pregnancy that sets the cardio-vascular disease clock ticking. The wrong kind of diet in the first few years of life can switch a child's metabolism towards metabolic syndrome later in life. Although we used to have the concept that a person's genes contain programmes that run the body and are 'fixed' to run so there's nothing you can do to change them, since the early 1990s there has been research into the effects of the environment on genes. Epigenetics is the study of how the environment that genes are exposed to can actually switch genes on and off – at a cellular level this is largely to do with what you eat and drink. This is called genetic expression; it isn't just an on/off switch but a process by which genes can be hyped up or dampened down.

The most important diet to feed yourself and infants is a low-GL diet – my Heart-friendly Diet – as explained in Chapter 21. (Pregnant women would also do well to follow this, see my book *Optimum Nutrition Before, During and After Pregnancy*; as would children, see *Optimum Nutrition for Your Child*.) The core principles are, in essence, the same for healthy children and healthy adults.

The environment is more important than the genes

What research is learning is that the environment to which we are exposed, especially the nutritional environment during foetal development and early life, but also throughout life, is as important as the genes we inherit. You can always, at considerable expense, have a genetic screen test to find out if you have any of the genes that would create a weakness in your biological matrix, so to speak. If the gene is active, the end result is that one of these markers, which I'll be discussing in detail later, will be raised – then you could take the appropriate action. If, for example, you have the genes that raise homocysteine, then why not measure your homocysteine and, if it is high, take more of the B vitamins that lower it? If you have the genes that raise lipoprotein(a) and LDL cholesterol and lower HDL, then why not measure these and, if high, take high-dose vitamin B_3 (niacin)? I will be explaining exactly what to measure, and what to do to lower your risk, whatever your genetic predisposition might be.

Even those with genetic predispositions, or inherited pre-dispositions due to a poor nutritional environment during foetal development, can decrease their risk through nutritional intervention. There *is* something positive that you can do to change the quality and length of your life.

How to get sick – guaranteed results

The good news is that after years of confusing, conflicting and complicated research and theories, we are starting to see some light at the end of the tunnel. A clear picture of how cardiovascular disease develops is emerging. With the knowledge of what you need to do to get heart disease, all you need do is flip the card to know how to prevent and reverse the situation.

The story starts before birth, ends with premature death and goes like this:

1   Inherit the genes that predispose you to producing lipoprotein(a) and homocysteine.

2   Be born short in length and skinny to a short, overweight mother, thereby developing insulin resistance.

3   Eat a refined-food diet deficient in vitamins C, B_3, B6, B12 and folic acid, thereby increasing lipoprotein(a) and homocysteine.

4   Expose yourself to plenty of oxidants from fried and burnt food, smoking, pollution and exhaust fumes.

15

5   Eat a diet deficient in antioxidant nutrients such as beta-carotene and vitamins C and E by avoiding fruit and vegetables, raw nuts and seeds.

6   Eat plenty of saturated fat from meat, dairy produce and non-free-range eggs and be deficient in essential fats from carnivorous fish, nuts and seeds.

7   Eat plenty of carbohydrates from sugar and refined foods.

8   Drink excess alcohol, avoid exercise, don't deal with your emotions and stay stressed. Also, eat when you are stressed.

9   Raise your blood pressure by eating salted and high-sodium foods, while avoiding fruits and vegetables, which are rich in important magnesium and potassium.

Do all this and you can reliably expect to have cardiovascular disease at a young age. On the other hand, eliminate these factors and you can expect to lead a long and healthy life, free from cardiovascular and other related diseases, adding at least ten years to your life, and improving its quality. Part 2 gives you a clear way to assess and reduce your risk.

The Holford low-GL diet put to the test

It is one thing to know what to do and another to do it. For this reason I set up some highly motivational groups across the UK and abroad, called Zest4Life. Run by registered nutritional therapists, the groups are attended by participants once a week for ten weeks, during which they learn how to start hardwiring good habits.

Ideally, these good habits mean a better diet, the right supplements, and exercise and lifestyle changes to reduce stress. We recently completed a 12-week project to assess the impact of the Zest4Life low-GL diet, including many of the key diet factors you'll be learning in this book, on a group of 21 patients at a GP surgery in Berkshire. All the participants had been identified as being at high risk of developing diabetes and/or heart disease, and exhibited one or more of the following risk factors (which are also a sign of metabolic syndrome, and I will be discussing this further in Chapter 3):

- Impaired fasting glucose

- Elevated glycosylated haemoglobin (HbA1c)

- Waist-to-hip ratio greater than 1 for men or 0.85 for women

- Elevated blood pressure

- Elevated LDL, and HDL and triglycerides outside the target range

Patients were encouraged to follow the low-GL eating plan and were supported in making lifestyle changes, including exercise and developing new habits. Nutritional supplements were not used, as we wanted to test the effects of the diet plus lifestyle changes alone. The clinical markers for chronic disease listed above were measured at the beginning of the programme and again at the end of 12 weeks, and weight and body composition were tracked during the 12 weeks.

The results speak for themselves. Everyone taking part lost weight and nine of the 21 participants lost over a stone (7kg). For the majority of participants, there was a clinically significant reduction in most of the markers. Not all these markers will make sense to you at this stage, but after you've finished reading Part 1 turn back and check out these results again.

Health markers	Before	After 12 weeks	Percentage improvement	Greatest individual change
Average weight	202lbs/ 14st 6lbs	187lbs/ 13st 5lbs	7.42%	- 31lbs 11.6%
Average HbA1C	6.9	5.9	14.5%	10.5–7.1 32.4%
Average fasting glucose	6.3	5.6	11.1%	9–6.2 31%
Average total cholesterol	5.27	4.59	12.9%	7.9–6.1 23%

Health markers	Before	After 12 weeks	Percentage improvement	Greatest individual change
Cholesterol/HDL ratio	4.12	3.69	8.7%	3.3–2 39%
Triglycerides	1.65	1.2	27%	5.4-1.2 77%
Blood pressure	137/81	131/73	4%/10%	128/88– 100/66 22%/25%
Triglyceride/HDL ratio	1.47	1.07	27%	5.4–1.14 78%

Case Study: Roger

In his own words Roger describes the experience and the results.

'Although I was not grossly overweight or particularly unfit, joining Patrick Holford's Zest4life group for a 12-week programme gave me the opportunity to exercise some control over the direction of travel of my own health, reducing my risk of obesity, heart disease, high blood pressure and diabetes – all associated with diet and exercise.

'The structure of weekly group meetings provided practical "bite size" knowledge of nutrition, supporting and justifying the changing of our eating habits and exercise routines. Being given weekly factual data of "outcomes/results" from the weight and body analysis machines was very motivational in monitoring the direct effects of the changes we were making. Clearly the level of motivation was directly proportional to the level of commitment individuals were able to make to change. Many of the improvements recorded in our blood results between the beginning and the end of the programme were truly impressive. For me personally the experience is potentially life changing and maybe even life saving. Before starting the programme I was eating what I thought was a reasonably healthy diet almost devoid of any processed foods, ready meals and takeaways so I was surprised that my risk of suffering heart disease and diabetes was much higher than I could reasonably have expected. This risk was reduced by half following the 12-week programme and in the process I lost nearly 1½ stone [9.5kg] in weight (from 16 stone 8 lbs [105.25kg] to 15 stone 2lbs [96kg]).

'What I found really convincing as a natural sceptic was the considerable lowering of blood pressure from 128/88 to 100/66 and other test results that showed a truly significant improvement, especially the reduction in triglycerides from 5.4 to 1.2 [a 78 per cent reduction] and HbA1c dropping from 6 per cent to 5.3 per cent [11.67 per cent]. Amazingly, these improvements were achieved purely by making relatively few changes to my eating habits and taking regular but moderate exercise involving walking and cycling. The only medication I had been taking prior to the programme was for hypertension, and as a result of my reduced blood pressure my doctor has reduced the dose by half, and he has commented that this is not a very common occurrence. I now have the knowledge and tools to continue to improve my overall health.'

Any drug that could produce these kinds of results would be an instant best-seller. Yet, here you see that small changes to your diet and exercise can make a massive difference to preventing and recovering from heart disease. As you'll see later, adding certain nutritional supplements can make a big difference, but they are supplements to a healthy diet, not a substitute for it. Sometimes it's necessary to have the support of a group of people or to see a nutritional therapist one-to-one, and I'll let you know how you can do this. But the first step to taking control of your heart health is to get informed. The rest of Part 1 explains the nature of the problem, and how your cardiovascular system works. Then, in Part 2, I'll examine the main keys to preventing and reversing heart disease.

CHAPTER 2

Understanding Blood Pressure and Pulse

Inside you is an amazing network of blood vessels which, if put end to end, would reach the moon! At their widest point these blood vessels measure 2.5cm (1in). At their narrowest point – the capillaries – they are only 1/400,000th of a centimetre. The cardiovascular system is made up of the heart and these blood vessels, which carry oxygen, fuel (in the form of glucose), building materials (amino acids), vitamins and minerals to every single cell in your body. Blood becomes oxygenated in the lungs where the tiny blood vessels (capillaries) absorb oxygen and then discharge carbon dioxide, which we breathe out. The oxygenated blood is then fed into the heart, which pumps it to all our cells. In the cells the blood vessels once more become a network of extremely thin capillaries through which oxygen and other nutrients pass.

Oxygen plus glucose is needed to make energy within every cell. The waste products are carbon dioxide and water, which pass from the cells into the capillaries. Blood vessels supplying cells with nutrients and oxygen are called arteries, while those that carry away waste products and carbon dioxide are called veins. Arterial blood is redder because oxygen is carried on a substance called haemoglobin, which contains iron, giving it a red tinge. The pressure in the arteries is also greater than in the veins. As well as returning to the heart, all blood passes through the kidneys, where waste products are removed and formed into urine, which is stored in the bladder ready for excretion.

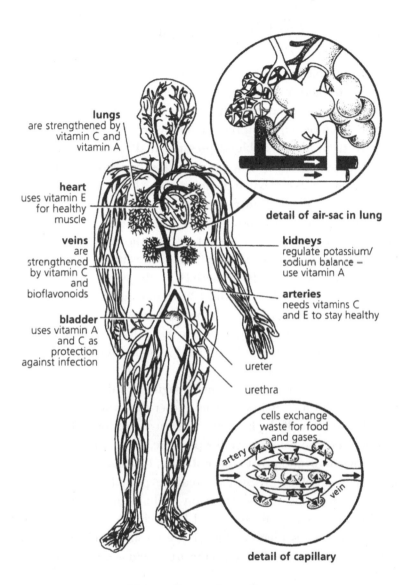

lungs
are strengthened by
vitamin C and
vitamin A

heart
uses vitamin E
for healthy
muscle

veins
are
strengthened
by vitamin C
and
bioflavonoids

bladder
uses vitamin A
and C as
protection
against infection

detail of air-sac in lung

kidneys
regulate potassium/
sodium balance –
use vitamin A

arteries
needs vitamins C
and E to stay healthy

ureter

urethra

cells exchange
waste for food
and gases

artery

vein

detail of capillary

The cardiovascular system

Blood pressure

One of the first signs of cardiovascular disease is increased blood pressure. To picture what happens, imagine a hosepipe attached to a tap that turns on and off. When the tap is on the pressure is greatest, and when the tap is off the pressure is lowest. That's what blood pressure is all about. A blood pressure of 120/80 means that the maximum pressure when the heart has just beaten is 120 units, and the minimum pressure when the heart is in a lull is 80 units. A blood pressure (also called BP) measurement consists of these two numeric readings. The first, written on top, is called systolic; the other, written underneath, is the more important diastolic, which measures the pressure when your heart is at rest. BP is measured in millimetres of mercury, written as 'mmHg' because HG is the symbol for mercury. A normal reading would be around 120/76 mmHg. If your blood pressure is above 140/90, you have hypertension – high blood pressure.

Approximately one in four people in the UK have hypertension, whereas only half the population have a blood pressure in the optimal range (below 120/80).

To understand what causes this, imagine that the hosepipe I used as an illustration earlier was metal rather than rubber. This would raise the pressure. If the hosepipe was furred up, or if the fluid was thicker, these too would raise the pressure. So raised blood pressure is a reliable indication that all is not right. Life-insurance companies rely heavily on blood pressure to predict expected lifespan.

The symptoms of hypertension include nosebleeds, tinnitus (ringing in the ears), dizziness and headaches – but you can easily have it without any obvious signs. Hypertension can be the result of any one of three main changes in the artery and is usually a combination of these:

Increased constriction The blood vessels contain a layer of muscle. If this muscle contracts too much the pressure increases. Smoking, caffeine and stress can cause this kind of constriction as can too much salt (sodium), or not enough magnesium, calcium or potassium. Insulin, the sugar hormone, also causes the kidneys to retain both water and salt, which then pushes up your blood pressure. This is because you have a greater volume of water in the blood, and because salt controls the balance between muscles contracting and relaxing. That's why balancing blood sugar, which reduces insulin, is critical for lowering blood pressure (see Chapter 8). When you're frightened or you're exercising you need your blood vessels to tense and narrow to pump more blood around the body, but then they should relax. When they stay tense for too long the result is high blood pressure – or hypertension. That's why stress is a major factor in heart disease, which I'll be discussing in Chapter 9.

Thicker blood If the blood is thicker, or stickier, this alone can cause small increases in blood pressure. The blood contains tiny plates, called platelets, which stick to each other. This ability to clot is what stops you bleeding to death if you cut yourself. Too much clotting, however, and you increase the risk of producing life-threatening blood clots, especially if the arteries are already narrow due to atherosclerosis.

Atherosclerosis This is a term that has come to mean a narrowing of a blood vessel due to damage and thickening of the blood vessel wall, often resulting in increased deposits of cholesterol and other substances. The blood vessel may also become more rigid and less elastic, increasing the pressure, much like the skin loses its elasticity with age. This can be caused by oxidation, fuelled by a lack of anti-oxidants, and also by sugar damage and raised homocysteine.

Blood pressure control is a complex, normally self-regulating system that is partly controlled by the ebb and flow of two pairs of minerals in and out of the cells lining the blood vessel walls. One of these pairs consists of sodium (salt) and potassium; sodium inside the cell pushes the pressure up, potassium inside brings it down. The other pair consists of calcium and magnesium – calcium raises while magnesium lowers. This explains why you're advised to keep your salt intake down (more sodium raises BP) and why one of the types of drug is a calcium channel blocker (keeping calcium out lowers BP). But it also highlights the way that two halves of the pairs are largely ignored by the conventional approach. As we'll see in Part 2, getting good amounts of potassium and magnesium in your diet or via a supplement is a sensible starting point for any blood pressure-lowering regime.

The body produces a potent antioxidant, nitric oxide (NO), to help promote healthy circulation and normal blood pressure. NO expands blood vessels, stops platelets clumping together, and reduces atherosclerosis, all of which helps control blood pressure. Many drugs work by mimicking or promoting NO; for example, a whiff of nitrogylcerine has an immediate, but short-term effect like NO. The famous Viagra drug, first introduced for cardiovascular health, promotes NO and hence circulation to the sex organs. It didn't prove sufficiently effective for heart disease. Later on we'll talk about nutrients that help promote NO.

Your ideal blood pressure and pulse

A blood pressure of 120/80 or less is ideal. A top figure (the systolic pressure) of more than 140, or a bottom figure (the diastolic pressure) of more than 90, indicates a potential problem. A blood pressure of 150/100 indicates a serious risk of heart disease; for example, a 55-year-old man with a blood pressure of 120/80 will, on average, live to the age of 78. A 55-year-old man with a blood pressure of 150/100 is predicted to live to 72. High blood pressure, or hypertension, is a silent killer. Only one in ten people with raised blood pressure are aware of it. After the age of 25 most people's blood pressure increases quite rapidly. So a yearly blood pressure check is always recommended. If you're healthy there's no reason why your blood pressure should increase with age. Many primitive cultures show no such rise.

What your pulse and blood-pressure readings indicate

	Low risk	Medium	High
Pulse	60–69	70–79	80+
Blood Pressure	90/60	126/86	136/90
	to	to	or
	125/85	135/89	higher

Your pulse rate, the number of heartbeats a minute, is less a measure of the health of your blood vessels and more an indication of the fitness of your heart; for example, a very fit cyclist may have a pulse rate of 40 whereas many people have a pulse rate of 80 beats per minute. So the cyclist's heart can get all the blood round the body with half the number of beats. His or her heart, which is essentially a muscle, is clearly stronger. The healthiest people have a pulse rate below 70 beats per minute. Interestingly, there is one lifespan statistic that is relatively consistent for all animals. We all have around 3 billion heartbeats in a life. It follows that if your pulse rate were 80, you would have a lifespan of 71 years, if it were 60, 95 years. The better your diet and exercise regime the lower your pulse will be.

Both your pulse and blood pressure can be lowered with optimum nutrition. A three-month trial on 34 people with high blood pressure at the Institute for Optimum Nutrition in London achieved an average 8-point drop in systolic and diastolic blood pressures, with the greatest decreases in those with the highest initial blood pressure.[6] Dr Michael Colgan found that, irrespective of age, people placed on comprehensive nutritional supplement programmes for five years had gradual decreases in blood pressure from an average of slightly above 140/90 to below 120/80.[7] Dr Colgan also found that their pulse rate dropped from an average of 76 to 65 over the five years.

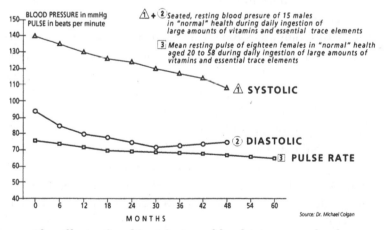

The effects of multinutrients on blood pressure and pulse

In Chapter 18 I'll show you how to put all these pieces together to lower your blood pressure to normal.

CHAPTER 3

Understanding Blood –
Cholesterol and Triglycerides

Most people think that eating too much fat and high-cholesterol foods blocks the arteries with cholesterol and that causes a heart attack. Every part of this sentence is untrue, as I will show you. Nevertheless, having a high cholesterol level is a risk factor for heart disease, but why your level goes high has almost nothing to do with eating cholesterol.

Cholesterol is a vital nutrient for both your body and brain, where it is most concentrated. The body actually makes cholesterol in the liver and we all carry approximately 150g (4¾oz) of it in our bodies. Of this, only 7g (¼oz) is carried in our blood. The body needs cholesterol to make sex and stress hormones and vitamin D and to digest and transport fats (lipids). It's also vital for brain function because it helps the brain cells to work properly. Cholesterol is not really the villain in relation to heart disease, but what happens to cholesterol is part of the problem.

Having said that, having a high blood cholesterol level, especially LDL cholesterol, is associated with a doubling of the risk of cardio-vascular disease. But it is the type of cholesterol in the body and the way the body clears the excess from the arteries that makes cholesterol relevant.

The ins and outs of cholesterol

Cholesterol is made in the liver and should return there after it has been released in bile into the digestive tract, where it helps to digest fats before being reabsorbed into the bloodstream. Certain protein 'ships', known as low-density lipoproteins (LDLs), have been found to be responsible for carrying cholesterol to the artery wall. Others, high-density lipoproteins (HDLs), help to return cholesterol to the

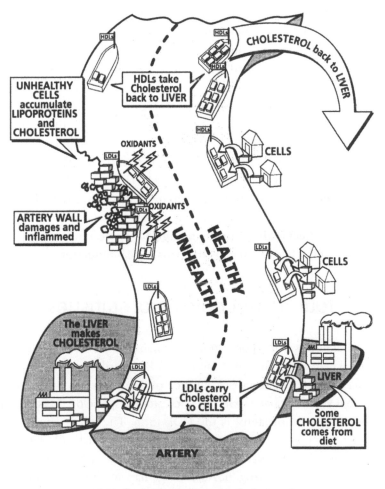

How the body transports cholesterol

liver. So if you have a low LDL cholesterol count and a high HDL cholesterol count, that is good news because it would mean that most of your cholesterol was on the HDL 'ship' that could remove it from the arteries. Actually, even LDL cholesterol is not all bad – we need some of it. But when there's too much it becomes particularly prone to oxidation and also glycation (a damaging process linked to too much sugar in the blood), and then the LDL particles don't look or function correctly. The immune system, your police force, 'arrests' them, engulfing them with cells called phagocytes, which then become full of fat and become 'foam' cells, which are found in the plaque of damaged arteries and are the main process that causes atherosclerosis.

HDL cholesterol is sometimes thought of as 'good cholesterol' and LDL cholesterol as 'bad cholesterol'. Because of this, the cholesterol test reports not only your overall cholesterol level, but also how much of that cholesterol is on the good HDL ship, and how much is on the bad LDL ship. If, for example, you have a high total cholesterol and much of it is in the form of LDL, your risk is high. Whereas if you have a low total cholesterol and much of it is on the HDL ship your risk is low. This is usually reported as the ratio of total cholesterol to HDL cholesterol. If it's 5:1 you have an average risk, if it's 8:1 you have a high risk and if it's 3:1 you have a low risk. Later on we'll examine the effect of drugs on changing your cholesterol statistics for the better, and what this means in terms of risk reduction.

Your ideal cholesterol statistics

Most laboratories will report a 'normal' range for total blood cholesterol of somewhere between 3 and 5mmol/l. Many cardiovascular experts, such as Dr Malcolm Kendrick, author of *The Great Cholesterol Con*, argue that you don't have to have a cholesterol level below 5, especially if more of your cholesterol is the HDL form. The upper level of the normal total cholesterol range used to be 6 and, statistically, having a level below this, between 5 and 6, doesn't increase risk. Some experts consider the ever-lowering 'normal' range has much more to do with widening the market for statin drugs than the evidence of any risk.

Although high cholesterol is considered a significant risk factor, low scores have, until recently, been ignored. Yet increasing evidence is linking low cholesterol levels to a number of mental and physical health problems. Among these are a hyperactive thyroid, certain cancers, suicidal and homicidal tendencies and mental illness. So there is a healthy balance – not too high, not too low. (Some cardiologists have the view that the lower your cholesterol the better and give strong drugs, statins, even to those with normal cholesterol levels. We will explore this idea in more detail in Chapter 6.)

Ideally, your HDL should be above 1.6mmol/l. If your HDL is below 1.04 mmol/l that's indicative of metabolic syndrome and a higher risk of heart disease.

One point to bear in mind is that so-called 'normal' cholesterol levels are based on people in average poor health. So what ranges exist in healthy people? This is the question Dr Emmanuel Cheraskin and colleagues set out to answer in a study on 1,281 doctors, using an accepted health rating scale, called the Cornell Medical Index (CMI), in which the participants complete a questionnaire asking health-related questions. In the entire group, they found a range of cholesterol scores between 2.8 and 13.5mmol/l. The healthiest people – those with a score of 0 on the CMI – had cholesterol levels between 4.6mmol/l and 6.2mmol/l.[8] In another study on dental students, Cheraskin measured the effects of eliminating refined carbohydrates and comparing it with the health of their gums. Those who achieved the best dental rating after dietary changes had cholesterol scores in the narrow band of 4.9 to 5.4mmol/l. I'd suggest that the healthiest cholesterol level is between 3.5 and 5.5mmol/l provided you've also got high HDL levels.

What your blood cholesterol level means

	Low Risk Mmol/l (UK)	Mg% (US)	Medium Mmol/l (UK)	Mg% (US)	High Mmol/l (UK)	Mg% (US)
Cholesterol	<5.18	200	6.2	240	>6.7	260
LDLs	<1.8	70	<2.6	100	>3.4	130
HDLs	>1.6	62	<1	39	<0.5	20
Cholesterol/HDLs	3:1		5:1		8:1	

Triglycerides – fats in the blood

Although nutritionists have been writing about the importance of triglycerides for several years, they have only recently been taken seriously as a major risk factor – perhaps more so than cholesterol. All fats, good and bad, are carried in the blood in the form of triglycerides. Sugar and alcohol can also be converted in the liver into fat, so they too can increase your level, as can eating too much fat, especially saturated fat. The fruit sugar, fructose, particularly, raises triglycerides.[9] The second biggest influence is a lack of omega fats. Increasing your intake of omega-3s (from fish, raw nuts and seeds) actually halves your triglyceride level so you need to have more omega-3 fats and fewer saturated or damaged trans-fats. (I'll go into this in much more detail in Chapter 7.)

An optimal triglyceride level is around 1mmol/l. You certainly don't want to have a level above 3.9 mmol/l, although, according to one study in the US, about a third of adults do, and the percentage is much higher among those who are both overweight and don't exercise.[10] Eating high-fat foods, such as red meat and dairy products, or a high-sugar or diet that is 'high GL' (meaning full of refined foods), especially if you have insulin resistance, raises your triglycerides, as does drinking too much alcohol.

Certain drugs, notably the contraceptive pill, steroid drugs (based on cortisone) and diuretics, given to lower blood pressure, can also increase triglycerides.

Triglycerides are normally tested as part of a routine medical and would be included in a standard medical screening. If you ask for a copy of your test results, this will be shown. If you've had your cholesterol measured, the chances are you will also have a result for your triglycerides. Ideally, your level should be below 1 mmol/l and certainly not above 2.5 mmol/l.

What your blood triglyceride level means

	Low Risk		Medium		High	
	Mmol/l (UK)	Mg% (US)	Mmol/l (UK)	Mg% (US)	Mmol/l (UK)	Mg (US)
Triglycerides	‹1	90	2.5	150	›2.5	100

Although triglycerides are now being increasingly recognised as an independent indicator of risk, there is much debate about whether or not triglycerides actually cause heart disease. It is certainly likely that having too many circulating blood fats puts pressure on the clearance systems, involving HDL, and may provide more unhealthy lipoproteins which can contribute to arterial damage and the development of plaques.

The perfect ratio – low triglycerides:high HDL

Probably the most predictive measure of all is your HDL-to-triglyceride ratio. This is because your triglycerides go higher in direct response to the excess fat you make if your blood sugar keeps going too high. This happens because the liver converts the excess glucose (or alcohol) from the blood into fat. As blood sugar spikes increase, the more LDL cholesterol and the less HDL cholesterol you have. This ratio is the most predictive of cardiovascular disease, so you should aim to get your ratio of triglycerides to HDL down to 3 or lower; for example, if your triglyceride level is 2 and your HDL level is 1, then you have a relatively low risk. For good health you want to have high HDL cholesterol and low triglycerides.

What your triglycerides:HDL level indicates

	Low Risk	Medium	High
Triglycerides:HDL	‹2:1	3	›4:1

Is your metabolism overheating?

Whether you already have heart disease or you are concerned about the possibility, or if you are overweight and not feeling great, there's a very good chance that your metabolism is already starting to shift into an unhealthy pattern which, when particularly pronounced, is called 'metabolic syndrome'. This is a precursor for both heart disease and type-2 diabetes. Heart disease is just one of a number of increasingly common health issues of the 21st century that are probably affecting you and members of your family, right now. And to get to the source of the problem it's important to recognise that good health means addressing the other health issues that are connected to it. Have a look at the illustration below; which diseases do you or your close circle of family and friends have? Many of those health issues were extremely rare a hundred years ago, so what has changed to make us more susceptible to them?

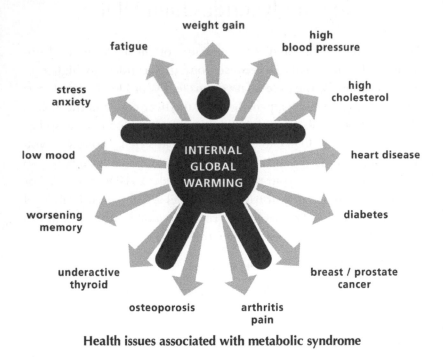

Health issues associated with metabolic syndrome

If you are suffering from what I call 'internal global warming' that means that you have metabolic syndrome. The cluster of problems illustrated above is being recognised more and more in mainstream medicine as metabolic syndrome, originally called 'syndrome x'. Since mainstream medicine prefers objective test results to nebulous 'subjective' symptoms, metabolic syndrome is officially diagnosed when you have three or more of the following:

- High blood sugar or glycosylated haemoglobin (above 5.7 per cent)

- High blood pressure (above 130/85)

- Increased waist circumference (above 102cm (40in) in men or 89cm (35in) in women)

- High triglycerides (above 3.9)

- Low HDL cholesterol (the 'good' cholesterol – below 1.03 in men and 1.3 in women)

- Insulin resistance

Many of these will be measured in a standard screening for cardiovascular health. You can also complete a free online Metabolic Check at www.patrickholford.com. This is part of an overall free check called the 100% Health Check. It will give you a better idea as to whether or not this is likely to be a problem for you.

An analysis of 87 studies involving almost a million people found that people with metabolic syndrome more than double their risk of developing cardiovascular disease, having a stroke or a heart attack or dying from it.[11] So it is important that you work on reversing this trend, and I am going to tell you how to do this in Parts 2, 3 and 4. The single biggest key is to eat a low glycemic load (low-GL) diet – my Heart-friendly Diet – which I explain in Chapter 8.

CHAPTER 4

The Red Herring of Cholesterol and Fat

Back in 1913 a Russian scientist, Dr Anitschkov, thought he had found the answer to heart disease: he found that it was induced by feeding cholesterol to rabbits. What he failed to realise, however, was that rabbits, being vegetarians, have no means for dealing with this animal fat.

Since the fatty deposits in the arteries of people with heart disease have also been found to be high in cholesterol, it was soon thought that these deposits were the result of an excess of cholesterol in the blood, possibly caused by an excess of cholesterol in the diet.

Such a simple theory had its attractions and many doctors still advocate a low-fat, low-cholesterol diet as the answer to heart disease, despite a consistent lack of positive results. In truth, this prevailing myth has been fuelled by the existence of highly profitable statin drugs, sold for their cholesterol-lowering ability, which are more easily marketed by making cholesterol the villain.

If the cholesterol theory were correct, we could expect that:

A   Eating lots of dietary cholesterol and fat would raise blood cholesterol and that people who do this would have a high incidence of heart disease;

B   Blood cholesterol levels would be good predictors of heart disease, and lowering blood cholesterol level would reduce the risk.

You would then have to prove that A leads to B, in other words that eating cholesterol raises cholesterol, which leads to heart disease.

Let's examine the evidence for the cholesterol theory, step by step, starting with whether or not eating cholesterol raises blood cholesterol.

Putting cholesterol to the test

An average egg contains about 275mg of cholesterol and two-thirds of its calories come from fat. So eggs are the perfect candidate for testing the theory that eating cholesterol, or high fat, raises blood cholesterol.

Dr Alfin-Slater, from the University of California, was one of the first, back in the 1970s, to test the cholesterol theory.[12] 'We, like everyone else, had been convinced that when you eat cholesterol you get cholesterol. When we stopped to think, none of the studies in the past had tested what happens to cholesterol levels when eggs, high in cholesterol, were added to a normal diet.'

He selected 50 healthy people with normal blood cholesterol levels. Half of them were given two eggs per day (in addition to the other cholesterol-rich foods they were already eating as part of their normal diet) for eight weeks. The other half were given one extra egg per day for four weeks, then two extra eggs per day for the next four weeks. The results showed no change in blood cholesterol. Later, Dr Alfin-Slater commented, 'Our findings surprised us as much as ever ...'

I've kept an eye on studies ever since and they all show the same thing: eating cholesterol doesn't raise blood cholesterol. Here's a more recent study from the University of Surrey in 2009. The researchers fed two eggs per day to overweight but otherwise healthy volunteers for 12 weeks while they simultaneously followed a reduced-calorie diet. A control group followed the diet but cut out eggs altogether.

Both groups lost between 3–4kg (6½–9lb) in weight and saw a fall in the average level of blood cholesterol.[13] Research leader, Professor Bruce Griffin, stated: 'When blood cholesterol was measured at both six weeks and twelve weeks, both groups showed either no change or a reduction, particularly in their LDL (bad) cholesterol levels, despite the egg group increasing their dietary cholesterol intake to around four times that of the control.'

But what if you've got a high blood cholesterol level already? A study from the University of Washington took 161 people with high cholesterol levels and fed them either two eggs a day or a cholesterol-free egg substitute. After 12 weeks those eating two eggs a day had a tiny non-significant increase in LDL cholesterol of 0.07mmol/l, and a significant increase in the 'good' HDL of 0.1mmol/l, and therefore no real change in the ratio of HDL to LDL cholesterol, which is the more important statistic.[14] To put this in context, if you turn to page 29 you'll see that having an LDL cholesterol below 1.8 is consistent with a low risk whereas having a level above 3.4 is consistent with a high risk. A tiny 0.07 increase is inconsequential.

What if there's something special about eggs? Other foods rich in cholesterol include shrimps. A more recent study from Rockefeller University gave participants either three servings (300g/10½oz) of shrimps or two large eggs a day, each providing 580mg of cholesterol. Researchers found that both groups had an increase in both the good HDL cholesterol and the less desirable LDL cholesterol, which they interpreted to mean that neither diet would be likely to make any significant difference to cardiovascular risk.[15]

Does eating high-cholesterol foods increase heart disease risk?

Surely eating lots of eggs or other high-cholesterol and high-fat foods must be bad news? The Inuit people of North America (Eskimos) were always an enigma with regard to the cholesterol theory. Their traditional diet, high in seal meat, has among the highest cholesterol levels of any cultural diet, yet their rate of cardiovascular disease is among the lowest. We now know, however, that their diet of seal meat is exceptionally high in omega-3 fats, which confer protection, as I'll explain in Chapter 7. But what about people eating high-cholesterol foods that aren't high in omega-3?

In fact, as long ago as 1974, a British advisory panel set up by the government to look at 'medical aspects of food policy on diet related to cardiovascular disease' issued this statement: 'Most of the dietary cholesterol in Western communities is derived from eggs, but we have found no evidence which relates the number of eggs consumed to heart disease.'[16]

Every study I've ever seen says the same thing. Study after study has repeatedly failed to find any increased risk of heart disease from eating six eggs a week.[17] One study finds that seven eggs or more a week confers a very slight increased risk but this is not confirmed by other studies, while two studies find that the risk is slightly higher in diabetics either eating lots of eggs or having a very high cholesterol intake in their diet.

It is now evident that there is no clear relationship between intake of dietary cholesterol and cardiovascular disease. How many millions of people have been avoiding eating eggs unnecessarily?

Having said this, however, a lot of high-cholesterol foods also happen to be high in saturated fat and are often also fried. Although this might not significantly raise cholesterol, you might get more oxidised cholesterol, which is bad news. It is therefore prudent not to go overboard on high-cholesterol foods, while at the same time there is no need for cholesterol phobia.

So if you are not diabetic you can assume that it is certainly safe to have six eggs a week. If you are diabetic it may be wise to limit your total cholesterol by having no more than three eggs a week and fewer other cholesterol-rich foods such as prawns, shrimps and shellfish; however, it is likely that if your overall diet is healthy, following the principles in this book, even this may be unnecessary.

Does eating a high-fat diet increase heart disease risk?

We've all been told to eat low-calorie low-fat diets, and supermarkets are full of low-fat foods that imply they can reduce your risk of heart disease.

There are a lot of inconsistencies in this subject in that some countries with a high fat intake (for example Finland) have a high rate of heart disease while others (like Greece) have a very low rate of heart disease. Then, of course, we have the Inuit, and also Pacific and other islanders who eat a large amount of coconut produce, high in saturated fat, and have a low risk of heart disease.

In 2010 the American Dietetic Association hosted the Great Fat Debate with top experts to explore these inconsistencies. One of these was Professor Walter Willetts from Harvard School of Public Health. He summarised the findings from decades of research.[18] For example, in 1989, the National Academy of Sciences concluded that the intake of total fat, independent of the relative content of different types of fatty acids, is not associated with high blood cholesterol levels and coronary heart disease. A review by the Food and Agricultural Organization, as well as a World Health Organization review, also states that there was no probable or convincing evidence for significant effects of total dietary fat on coronary heart disease.[19] However, if you do eat less fat you are also going to be eating more of something else, and what you replace it with makes all the difference. According to Willetts, 'If you replaced saturated fat with polyunsaturated fat there was a reduction in risk [of heart disease]. But if you replaced total fat or saturated fat with carbohydrate, no reduction in risk [was found].' In Chapter 7 you'll see that increasing omega-3 fats, which are the most polyunsaturated, reduces your risk, while increasing your carbohydrate load, explained in Chapter 8, quite dramatically increases your risk and also raises both cholesterol and blood fats (triglycerides).

The same conclusion is reached in a study of studies: a meta-analysis in the *American Journal of Clinical Nutrition* reports that 'an independent association of saturated fat intake with cardiovascular disease risk has not been consistently shown in prospective epidemiologic studies'. Replacement of saturated fat by polyunsaturated or monounsaturated fat lowers both LDL and HDL cholesterol; however, replacement with a higher carbohydrate intake, particularly refined carbohydrate, can exacerbate many risk factors for cardiovascular disease including the 'atherogenic dyslipidemia associated with insulin resistance and obesity, increased triglycerides, small LDL particles, and reduced HDL cholesterol'.[20]

In other words, if you eat a diet high in sugar and refined carbohydrates not only are they converted into fat but they also raise cholesterol, whereas slow-releasing carbs, high in soluble fibres, such as oats, reduce risk. In Chapter 17 you'll also learn about other cholesterol-lowering foods, including beans.

So, even though I have shown you that dietary fat per se, and cholesterol in particular, does not increase your risk of heart disease, switching from a high animal-protein diet towards more fish and vegetable protein, especially soya, does have significant effects in terms of lowering both blood cholesterol and fat levels, as well as reducing heart disease risk.

Cholesterol is more a marker than a cause

Although you've seen that eating cholesterol and fat does not raise either blood cholesterol or heart disease risk, you'll find out that foods that tend to reduce cardiovascular risk do tend to lower cholesterol levels as well. So your blood cholesterol statistics are not irrelevant, they are just not quite as important as we've been led to believe. According to Professor Meir Stampfer from Harvard School of Public Health 'total cholesterol is not a great predictor of risk'. His research group finds that eating a low-carb (low-GL) diet is one of the best ways of both reducing risk and lowering cholesterol.

If you or your doctor rely only on cholesterol to predict risk without assessing other critical risk factors such as triglycerides, homocysteine, glycosylated haemoglobin and lipoprotein(a), you may still be at high risk despite a normal cholesterol level. A massive US survey of 136,905 patients found that more than half of those hospitalised for a heart attack had perfectly normal cholesterol levels (LDL below 2.6mmol/l), according to National Institute of Clinical Excellence and Department of Health guidelines which recommend an LDL below 3mmol/l. Seventeen per cent had healthy cholesterol levels (LDL below 1.8mmol/l).[21]

A five-year survey of elderly people aged 85 found that cholesterol was also a very poor predictor of cardiovascular death several years later. The best predictor by far is your homocysteine level. If a person's homocysteine level was above 13, it predicted no less than two-thirds of all deaths five years on.[22] (More on this in Chapter 10.)

You certainly don't want to put all your eggs in the cholesterol basket, because you might miss other important indicators. If you do have a high cholesterol level, however, avoiding cholesterol foods isn't going to make much difference. But there are other diet and lifestyle changes that will.

The reason for this is that the body needs cholesterol and makes what it needs. It is only when you are eating, or living, in such a way that stops the normal cycle of cholesterol production and clearance by HDL that you start to get a change in cholesterol statistics; for example, if you eat a lot of fried foods or smoke (both of which are high in oxidants) and eat very few vegetables (which are high in antioxidants) cholesterol can become damaged by oxidation. Then the immune system attacks it, producing harmful foam cells. Alternatively, if you eat a high-sugar or high-GL diet, you start making more insulin, and both the high sugar and insulin damage cholesterol particles that start to accumulate. Also, the excess sugar is converted into fat, and up go your triglycerides (blood fats). Also, those soluble fibres in low-GL foods help to eliminate excess cholesterol. So the wrong kind of diet means you have more garbage and less efficient waste disposal, which is reflected by raised LDL and lowered HDL.

It's not just about diet, though. In Chapter 9 you'll find out that stress (and exercise) also plays a major part in raising heart disease risk and cholesterol.

It is not really the cholesterol per se that causes the damage that leads to arterial disease, but that high LDL and low HDL cholesterol is a predictive marker, or an indicator, that you are eating the wrong kind of diet or living too stressful a life.

If you take a statin drug that blocks the enzyme in the liver that makes cholesterol it is a no brainer that cholesterol levels will come down. After all, the brain and body need cholesterol to stay healthy. So, in effect, your liver and brain, when starved of cholesterol by taking these drugs, are going to suck every bit of available cholesterol out of the blood for use elsewhere. While these drugs do slightly reduce the risk in those who have heart disease it is highly likely that the mechanism by which they do this involves their anti-inflammatory effects,[23] rather than because they lower cholesterol per se. Lowering cholesterol is more likely to be a side effect, and a bad one at that.

Why low cholesterol is as bad for you as high cholesterol

Some people never give up and there's talk that we just need to lower cholesterol even more to get more benefit from these rather ineffectual drugs – as if the lower your cholesterol is the better.

All the talk of aggressively lowering cholesterol tends to ignore just how vital it is for the smooth running of our bodies; for example, it helps to repair damaged arteries, it is the raw material for making sex hormones, it is vital for laying down memories in the brain and for the proper working of the body's communication chemicals, called neurotransmitters.[24]

So it's hardly surprising that blocking the production of cholesterol in the liver, which is what statins do, causes all sorts of problems. Many of these are simply the problems that happen when you have too low cholesterol, but some are the consequence of statins knocking out the essential nutrient CoQ_{10}.

When you realise that cholesterol is a vital nutrient for the brain and body, it makes no sense to lower it beyond healthy levels (between 4 and 6mmol/l, provided your HDLs are reasonably high). But could low cholesterol be bad for you? Here are a few facts you might want to know:

Having too low a cholesterol level increases the risk of stroke Japan used to have a very low fat intake in the 1950s, and average cholesterol levels of 3.9mmol/l, but it also had a very high number of people suffering haemorrhagic strokes (that's the worst kind; see Chapter 5 for a full explanation of strokes).[25] After following advice to increase fat intake, largely from animal protein, their cholesterol levels went up to an average of 4.9mmol/l by 1999, and their stroke risk went down. In the last 50 years stroke risk (both haemorrhagic and ischaemic) has reduced by 600 per cent.

Having too low cholesterol increases risk of death Once you are getting below 4mmol/l risk of death actually increases. The danger of having too low cholesterol seems strongest in older people, say over the age of 60. This association is made clear in Dr Malcolm Kendrick's book *The Great Cholesterol Con* if you'd like to dig deeper.

Having too low cholesterol is also associated with increased rates of depression and suicide According to a study of 121 healthy young women by Duke University psychologist Edward Suarez, low cholesterol is a potential predictor for depression and anxiety.[26] An eight-year Finnish study of 29,000 men aged 50–69, published in the *British Journal of Psychiatry*, found that those reporting depression had significantly lower average blood cholesterol levels than those who did not, despite a similar diet.[27] One possible reason is that vitamin D is made from cholesterol and, as we will see in Part 2, exposure to sunlight converts cholesterol in the skin into vitamin D.

Having too low cholesterol is associated with feeling more aggressive This association is thought to be because not having enough cholesterol disrupts serotonin, a key brain neurotransmitter required for balancing your mood.[28] Having a low HDL has the strongest association.

None of this should be at all surprising if you recognise cholesterol for what it is: a vital nutrient, and a relatively poor marker for heart disease – certainly not the principal cause. It is extraordinary how much emphasis has been put on it, and its treatment with rather ineffective cholesterol-lowering drugs, as I'll show you in Chapter 6.

So what does cause heart disease, and how do you reverse it? That's what Part 2 is about, starting with the need to eat more fat of the right kind: essential omega-3 fats.

CHAPTER 5

Defining Heart Disease and Understanding Your Diagnosis

Any disease of the blood vessels is called cardiovascular disease. More popularly it's known as 'heart disease', although this is slightly misleading because cardiovascular disease can occur in the brain too, resulting in a blockage there which can cause a stroke (see below). This is known as cerebrovascular disease (cerebro = brain). Blockages can also occur in the legs and other parts of the body, in which case they are known as thrombosis. But the most common site of blockage is in the coronary arteries, which actually feed the heart itself with blood. This is called coronary artery disease. About half of all deaths from cardiovascular disease are from coronary heart disease and a quarter are from strokes.

The main life-threatening diseases are diseases of the arteries. Over a number of years, changes can occur within the artery walls that lead to deposition of unwanted substances, including cholesterol, other fats and calcium. These deposits are called arterial plaque, or atheroma from the Greek word *athērē* for groats (porridge), because of their porridge-like consistency. The presence of arterial deposits and thickening is called atherosclerosis. Atherosclerosis occurs in very particular parts of the body, as shown on page 45. Atherosclerosis, coupled with thicker blood containing blood clots, can lead to a blockage in the artery, stopping blood flow. If this occurs in the arteries feeding any part of the heart, that section of the heart dies from a lack of oxygen. This is called a myocardial infarction, or heart attack. Before this occurs many people are diagnosed as having angina, a condition in which there is a limited supply of oxygen to the heart due to partial blockage of coronary arteries, characterised by chest pain, usually on exertion or when under stress.

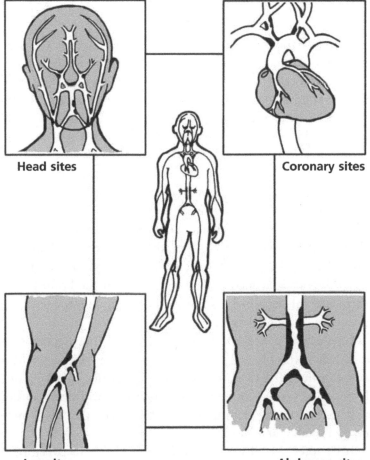

Head sites

Coronary sites

Leg sites

Abdomen sites

Common atherosclerotic sites

Understanding strokes

Stroke affects around 150,000 people in the UK each year.[29] It is the third most common cause of death in England and Wales,[30] responsible for over 50,000 deaths a year.[31] Although most people think that stroke affects only middle-aged or older men, women, young adults and children can all be affected. In fact, stroke accounts for 13 per cent of deaths in women in the UK[32] and although men are more likely to suffer a stroke, women are more likely to die from one.

A stroke happens when there is a disturbance in the brain's blood supply, which starves cells of oxygen and leads to cell death and a loss of brain function. There are two main types of stroke: ischaemic and haemorrhagic. Ischaemic strokes are more common and occur when blood flow to or within the brain is blocked. This blockage could happen for a variety of reasons. A blood clot might form in one of the four main arteries carrying blood to the brain (the right and left carotid arteries, and the right and left vertebro-basilar arteries) or in smaller arteries and capillaries within the brain. Alternatively, a blood clot, fat globule or air bubble present in a blood vessel in another part of the body could be carried to the brain. Haemorrhagic strokes are the type where a damaged or weakened artery bursts and there is bleeding into the brain. These damaged blood vessels could be located within the brain (causing an intracerebral haemorrhage) or on the brain surface (causing a subarachnoid haemorrhage).

The effects of a stroke differ simply because they depend on the area in which the blockage occurs and the size of artery affected. A stroke in the left half of the brain will affect the right side of the body and vice versa. Blockage of a main artery will result in much more damage than the blockage of a small capillary that only supplies blood to a smaller area of the brain.

(In Chapter 20 I'll explain how to maximise recovery from a stroke.)

Thrombosis, claudication, embolisms and aneurisms

If a blockage occurs in the legs, this can result in leg pain, which is a form of thrombosis (a thrombus is a blood clot). When peripheral arteries become blocked this can result in poor circulation in the feet or hands and, eventually, pain and lameness. This is called claudication. Sometimes a blood clot or a part of plaque dislodges and gets stuck, causing a lack of blood supply to an area of the body. This is called an embolism and can result in a stroke or heart attack. Sometimes, in a weakened artery with high pressure, often caused by arterial blockages, a rupture occurs with a balloon-like bubble of blood forming. This is called an aneurism. If this bursts it can lead to, for example, a cerebral haemorrhage, if it is located in the main arteries leading to the brain.

Congenital defects

A small percentage of heart disease is caused by defects that are already there at birth. These are called congenital defects and may affect a valve in the heart or result in an artery that is too narrow. These defects cannot be corrected by changes in diet and lifestyle and may require surgical intervention. But many minor congenital defects, such as very small holes in the heart between the chambers, do not have any impact on health; however, coupled with decreasing cardiovascular health, they may represent a point of weakness.

How heart attacks happen

The common misunderstanding about heart attacks is that arteries become blocked by hardened deposits, rich in calcium and cholesterol. Although calcified plaques do develop in the arteries they rarely cause a heart attack.

Instead, it appears that the real danger is from soft, vulnerable plaque, which develops because the unhealthy arteries trigger a state of inflammation, which alerts the immune system to clean up the mess. Immune cells called macrophages start gobbling up damaged LDL particles, and become foam cells, which are a main component of fatty streaks in the arteries. As part of the inflammatory process smooth muscle cells grow over the foam cells forming a fibrous cap. If this cap breaks (as part of an inflammatory process), the contents spill out into the bloodstream and can produce a blockage downstream, leading to a heart attack or stroke.

This is why it is not good to have too much LDL cholesterol or triglycerides in the blood. Also, you should not have too much homocysteine (which can directly damage the arteries) or too much inflammation.

A key measure of inflammation is something called C-reactive protein, or CRP for short. This is being increasingly measured as an indicator of cardiovascular risk and inflammation. (There is also an even better test called 'high sensitivity CRP' or hsCRP.)

Systems medicine and metabolic syndrome

Many of the key interventions for reducing cardiovascular risk – a low-GL diet, adequate omega-3 fats, more antioxidant nutrients such as vitamin C, more soluble fibre, as well as statin drugs and aspirin – all reduce inflammation. So, rather than conceiving of heart disease as a 'plumbing' problem, with too much fat and cholesterol as the gunk, there's a new concept emerging of cardiovascular disease as a systemic problem, with increased inflammation, poor glycation (sugar imbalance), poor methylation (with raised homocysteine and a lack of B vitamins) and poor lipidation (a lack of anti-inflammatory omega-3s and vitamin D). In my book *The 10 Secrets of 100% Healthy People* these are the main underlying processes that determine whether or not you are going to stay healthy.

Of course, this more systems-based way of thinking, perhaps akin to 'internal global warming', makes it increasingly obvious that the solution is unlikely to be a drug that simply blocks some pathway, be it the production of cholesterol, or calcium entering into cells to lower blood pressure. The solution, instead, has to be about reversing global warming, which means changing the set of circumstances that created the problem in the first place – diet, stress, lack of exercise and so on.

Increasingly, a systems-based way of approaching heart disease has focused on identifying a biological shift towards metabolic syndrome. Metabolic syndrome is not a disease as such, in the way that heart disease is, but a cluster of symptoms, diseases and test results that indicate a change in one's metabolic processes.

If you don't have heart disease but your health is not good you could well have metabolic syndrome; if you are currently suffering from heart disease, or have had a heart attack or stroke, you almost certainly do have metabolic syndrome. This is especially true if you also have a number of the other symptoms or health issues shown in the illustration 'Health issues associated with metabolic syndrome' on page 32.

Before we start looking at the key factors, and processes, that tip your body into a state of inflammation and metabolic syndrome, the next chapter explains the more common drugs on offer, what they target, how effective they are, and also their downsides. In my view, while drugs can be life saving in the short-term, the only long-term solution is to undo the damage.

CHAPTER 6

The Truth About Cardiovascular Drugs

By now, armed with a reasonable understanding of the dynamics of cardiovascular disease, we can examine the overall scale of benefit and potential harm from the most commonly prescribed cardiovascular drugs. There are several categories of heart medications, each designed to affect the different aspects of cardiovascular health that are measured. The main ones are:

- Cholesterol-lowering drugs, including statins
- Blood pressure-lowering drugs, including thiazides (diuretics), beta blockers, ACE inhibitors, calcium channel blockers, and nitrovasodilators
- Blood-thinning drugs to make clotting less likely, such as warfarin (coumadin) and aspirin

If you have cardiovascular disease or are at a high risk of developing it, the chances are you're on more than one of these medications already. All of them interfere with some aspect of your body's chemistry and none are necessary if you address the underlying causes of heart disease; however, having said that, please do not change your medication without consulting your doctor.

Statins and cholesterol-lowering drugs

About a third of all money spent on cardiovascular drugs is spent on statins. The big brands include Simvastatin, Atorvastatin, Pravastatin,

Rosuvastatin and Fluvastatin. If you've had a heart attack or have significant cardiovascular risk, research published in 2003 showed that statins can reduce your risk of a heart attack by up to 60 per cent, and your risk of stroke by 17 per cent.[33] However, the risk reduction is minimal in the first year you take it. If you haven't had a heart attack but your cholesterol level is above 5mmol/l, you'll probably be prescribed a statin. But are they worth taking?

At first sight, this might seem like a wise precaution. But not everyone agrees. If you haven't had a heart attack, taking statins 'does not significantly reduce all causes of mortality or the overall risk of serious illness', according to Dr John Abramson of the clinical medical faculty at Harvard Medical School. Almost half of people diagnosed as needing statins didn't need them at all. This was determined by actually scanning their arteries for plaque. A quarter of the patients deemed as needing statins had no detectable plaque at all.[34]

Overall, statin medication can be expected to lower LDL cholesterol by an average of 3.8mmol/l if taken for several years. Statins, however, are not very effective at raising HDL cholesterol, which is the more important indicator of reducing your risk (see Chapter 4) and the one that can be most influenced by changing your diet.

For over a decade there has been a worldwide marketing campaign to heavily promote these rather ineffective drugs. At the height of statin fever there was even talk of putting them in the water supply. 'If we can give them a pill in their 30s or 40s, their chances of having a heart attack will be slashed. It could be given to healthy people as a supplement to prevent their arteries becoming clogged,' read one newspaper front page in 2006.[35] In July 2007, the UK government heart disease supremo, Professor Roger Boyle, declared that blanket prescribing of statins to all those over 50 would have the biggest effect on saving lives. UK GPs are financially rewarded to test cholesterol, and lower it, and are encouraged to prescribe statins to anyone with a cholesterol level over 5mmol/l.

While the mainstream view is that statins benefit virtually everyone, there is good reason to believe that if you are a man aged over 69, or a woman of any age, they are not going to do you much good.

It's worth making a distinction here between taking them to cut your chances of having another heart attack (secondary prevention) – when they do work – and taking them to lower your risk of a heart attack when you haven't had one (primary prevention). About 75 per cent of people on statins get them for primary prevention.

Just how poor the evidence is and how little effort has been made to discover how many people are troubled by side effects was highlighted by a review of statins by the respected Cochrane Collaboration at the beginning of 2010. It analysed trials involving 34,272 people who hadn't had a heart attack and found little evidence that taking a statin would protect people from having a first heart attack unless their risk was classified as high. One trial gave 42,800 people with no history of cardiovascular events statins or placebos. After almost four years on the drugs there was no change in risk of death, even from cardiovascular disease, but there was a small reduction in heart attack risk of 1.7 per cent. This equates to one person in 60 taking the drug who would be saved from having a non-fatal heart attack.[36]

These are drugs given to about four and a half million healthy people in the UK, but researchers say that if you are over 65 or female the evidence isn't even as strong as stated above, because most of the trials involved white, middle-aged males, so the results don't necessarily apply to anyone else.

Statins won't lengthen your life

Even if the evidence that statins cut the risk of having a heart attack is weak, surely they prevent people dying early from a heart attack? Unfortunately not. A study in the *Lancet* in 2007 found that even though the drugs prevented a few heart attacks, none of the patients lived any longer as a result. That's bad enough – if you are told this pill will cut your risk of a heart attack, you assume that it will also make you live longer – but it gets worse. Men over 69 didn't benefit from taking statins at all – they didn't live longer and didn't have fewer heart attacks – and women of any age didn't benefit either.[37]

According to the study's author, Harvard professor John Abramson, you do benefit a bit if you have a high risk (for example, if you have high cholesterol or are overweight) and you're aged between 30 and 69 years. But the amount is hardly impressive. Fifty people have to be treated for five years to prevent just one event involving the heart. A more recent study on many more people, so the results could be expected to be more accurate, came up with figures for reduction in mortality that were even less impressive.

The study analysed trials involving 65,000 people who also didn't have heart disease but just a raised risk and found that out of 10,000 people who took the drugs for nearly four years just seven would avoid dying from any cause including heart disease.[38] 'The number of deaths prevented didn't reach statistical significance,' said lead researcher Professor Kausik Ray of St George's Hospital in South London. 'That means it could have happened by chance.' Yet this study and the Cochrane one have made barely a dent in prescribing.

Another trial gave statins versus placebo to patients with heart failure for just under four years. Those on statins had no reduction in risk.[39] According to the lead researcher, Dr Philip Poole-Wilson from Imperial College, London, 'The results should humble researchers and remind them that medical decisions should be guided by science, and not strongly held opinion.' Another group in this trial received omega-3 fish oils and *did* reduce their risk.

Suppose you are a woman with a very high risk of heart disease, how much benefit could you expect from taking statins? To answer this question for the GP magazine *Pulse*, Dr Malcolm Kendrick (author of *The Great Cholesterol Con*) analysed a major statin trial called HPS – which is frequently quoted as showing that statins benefit women – and concluded that if you took statins for 30 years, you would gain, on average, just one extra month of life.

What if you're a man? A trial involving 45,000 men deemed at high risk, with an average cholesterol level of 7mmol/l, most with pre-existing angina, treated over an average of 15 years, resulted in 57 added life years divided among the 45,000 men.[40] So, if you treated someone for 30 years, you could expect $\frac{1}{26}$th of a year of extra life: about two weeks.

The downside of statins

Besides the fact that a large number of people have to take a statin for just one of them to benefit, there's another problematic feature of statins – that is, the side effects.

Your doctor is unlikely to mention that as well as blocking LDL cholesterol, statins also reduce production of an enzyme known as co-enzyme Q_{10} (CoQ_{10}), which is, ironically, essential for heart health. A deficiency in CoQ_{10} has been associated with fatigue, muscle weakness and soreness, and heart failure.[41]

Just how serious these problems are is still unclear, not least because the major trials of statin drugs excluded those with class 3 and 4 heart failure, a major effect of CoQ_{10} deficiency.[42] (For more on CoQ_{10}, see Chapter 12.)

The Cochrane review on statins lists the recorded side effects as cataracts, acute kidney failure, and moderate or severe liver dysfunction along with sleep disturbances, memory loss, sexual dysfunction, depression, and (very rarely) interstitial lung disease. Common symptoms associated with statins include dizziness, headache, extreme fatigue, swelling of the ankles, muscle aches, fatigue and suppressed immunity. They also increase your risk of diabetes.

Even though the drugs have been prescribed to millions for over a decade, the reviewers found that the trials don't give nearly enough information about side effects. Over half the trials didn't report on adverse events at all, and they noted that there had been no attempt to assess the risk of some potentially serious side effects such as cognitive impairment (brain fog, as some patients call it), transient amnesia or the very real risk of diabetes when cholesterol is lowered too fast.[43] The case of NASA astronaut Duane Graveline is an interesting one. He was prescribed statins after a heart attack. After six weeks on the drug he lost his memory for six hours. Later, he lost it completely for 12 hours.[44] Although this side effect is quite rare, there are many other reports of memory loss caused by statins.

Your doctor will very likely tell you about the risks of muscle pain and weakness (myopathy) and a harmful change in liver function, although he/she will say they are very rare. But, again, that might not be the whole story. One study in the *British Medical Journal* found that when 22 professional athletes with very high cholesterol levels were put on statins, 16 of them stopped the treatment because of the side effects.[45] Competitive athletes are known to be more sensitive to muscle pain than other people.

Case Study: Fiona

With a cholesterol level of 8.5mmol/l, Fiona was prescribed atorvastatin.

> 'I only took one tablet and woke up at 3.00am with pins and needles, which gradually crept up my arms and across my face and tongue. Next morning I felt as if someone had punched me in the right shoulder.'

They certainly don't suit everybody. Instead, Fiona opted for the natural approach – diet, exercise and stress control – and managed to lower her cholesterol to 4.4mmol/l.

The frequency of side effects is downplayed

One of the reasons the studies for side effects, which doctors rely on, report low levels is because people who have any illness or who don't respond well are excluded from the trials. The same *British Medical Journal* article outlined above found that in one recent big trial – used to show how safe statins are – almost half the 18,000 people recruited to begin with weren't included. Of course, in the real world those are just the sort of people who would be given them. And this doesn't begin to estimate the effect of adding a statin if you are already taking a number of other drugs.

There is another reason why official adverse drug reaction (ADR) figures for statins are very low: when patients say the drugs are having a bad effect, doctors don't believe them. Whereas 98 per cent of 650 patients surveyed reported a foggy mental state, only 2 per cent of their doctors accepted it could be linked with taking statins. The figures for nerve pains in hands and feet (96 per cent vs. 4 per cent believed) and muscle pain (86 per cent vs. 14 per cent) were equally bad.[46]

Even more worrying is the question mark hanging over a possible link between statins and cancer.[47] They certainly give cancer to laboratory animals, and one of the big trials, called Prosper, which involved elderly patients, found taking statins raised your risk. This was dismissed at the time because no other trials had found it. But because cancer is much more likely to occur in older patients and because Prosper is the only trial undertaken on older patients, it's quite possible that fewer patients had heart attacks but developed cancer instead.[48]

Take coenzyme-Q_{10} if you're on a statin – and if you're not

If you have decided to take statins because you have already had a heart attack or because you are at high risk and feel it is worth it anyway, you really ought to take a supplement of CoQ_{10}. That's because as well as reducing cholesterol production in the liver, statins also interfere with this vital antioxidant. Among other things, it is vital for proper functioning of the mitochondria (the power plants in every cell). There's plenty of evidence to suggest that this could explain why muscle fatigue and pain are major side effects of statins. But it also raises concerns about putting extra stress on the heart, which uses a huge amount of CoQ_{10}. The severity of heart failure correlates with people who have the lowest levels. In a small study, 10 out of 14 subjects with no history of heart problems developed heart rhythm abnormalities when given statins, whereas giving CoQ_{10} reversed the abnormality in 8 out of 9.[49]

Research in America has shown that a high-dose CoQ_{10} supplement can reverse muscle pains. Fifty patients who had been on statins for two years were taken off the drug because they were complaining of muscle pains and other side effects. Giving them CoQ_{10} dramatically improved their symptoms.[50] Like others, the scientist in this trial commented that statin-related side effects were much more common than the big studies show. He also found that taking the patients off statins didn't make their blocked-up arteries any worse. A warning on statin packets is now mandatory in Canada, saying that CoQ_{10} reduction 'could lead to impaired cardiac function in patients with borderline congestive heart failure', but this warning is not added in the UK or Ireland.

If on statins, you need at least 90mg a day of CoQ_{10} (although speak to your doctor if you are taking blood-thinning medication). Furthermore, there are also many good reasons to supplement CoQ_{10} if you have heart disease, which I'll tell you about in Chapter 14. An alternative to statins, which lowers cholesterol just as well, but raises HDL cholesterol far better, is high-dose niacin (vitamin B_3), which I'll be talking about in Chapter 11. Very importantly though, don't mix statins with high-dose, sustained-release niacin, as evidence collected in the prematurely suspended AIM-HIGH clinical trial suggests there is no positive effect on cardiovascular events and there may be a small increased risk of ischaemic stroke.[51]

Blood pressure-lowering drugs

Of all the cardiovascular medicines, more prescriptions are written out for blood pressure-lowering drugs than for any other kind – around 40 million a year.[52] These drugs fall into five main categories, described below, but all of them produce similar reductions in blood pressure – a drop of around 5.5mmHg in diastolic blood pressure. In fact, there has been a big debate in the last few years about whether the newer, expensive ACE inhibitors are actually any better than the older, very cheap diuretics, following a major trial published in 2002 that found no difference between them.[53]

Whatever their relative merits, all these blood pressure-lowering drugs come with considerable risks, a fact that has been known by doctors for years. One of the first proper controlled trials, for instance, was done over 20 years ago on the diuretics. Nicknamed MRFIT (Multiple Risk Factor Intervention Trial), it involved 12,800 men at high risk of heart attack because they smoked and had high cholesterol and high blood pressure. The trial compared 'usual care' with the aggressive use of diuretics and found that even though diuretics did lower blood pressure, not only was there no reduction in risk of death among those being more aggressively treated, those with borderline hypertension (below 150/100) had a higher risk of death.[54]

Thiazides

These drugs are diuretics that essentially work by telling your kidneys to make you urinate more, as less liquid in the blood equals less pressure. They include chlorothiazide, benzthiazide and cyclothiazide. Of course, as soon as you increase the flow of urine, a number of vital minerals get washed out of the body as well so you can end up with too little potassium and magnesium. Some types of drugs spare potassium, including spironolactone and triamterene, but not the vital heart mineral magnesium. Also, lowering the amount of fluid in the blood causes the body to retain more sodium. So this kind of approach is fighting against the body's design and makes no sense over the long term.

Side effects Kidney damage, fatigue, muscle cramping, faintness and an increased incidence of gallstones. Long-term use may increase cholesterol and the risk of heart irregularities and blood sugar levels, so they're especially bad news for both full-blown and borderline diabetics.

The longer you are on these drugs, the greater the risks become. Since blood pressure can be relatively easily lowered by dietary and lifestyle changes, it makes sense to do these first before incurring all the potential hazards of these medications. As an editorial in a 1991 issue of the *British Medical Journal* stated:

> Treatment of hypertension is part of preventive medicine and like all preventive strategies, its progress should be regularly reviewed by whoever initiates it. Many problems could be avoided by not starting antihypertensive treatment

until after prolonged observation. Patients should no longer be told that treatment is necessarily for life: the possibility of reducing or stopping treatment should be mentioned at the outset.[55]

ACE inhibitors

These drugs block an enzyme (known as angiotensin-converting enzyme) that is necessary for the production of a substance that causes blood vessels to tighten. As a result, they relax blood vessels, lowering blood pressure. ACE inhibitors have names that usually end in 'pril', such as captopril, ramipril and trandolapril.

Side effects There are plenty of them with these drugs: a dry and persistent cough, headache, diarrhoea, loss of taste, nausea, unusual tiredness, dizziness, light-headedness or fainting, skin rash with or without itching, fever and joint pain. ACE inhibitors are contra-indicated if you are pregnant, and not suitable for those with kidney or liver problems. They can cause excess potassium accumulation, the symptoms of which are confusion, irregular heartbeat, nervousness, numbness or tingling in hands, feet or lips, shortness of breath or difficulty breathing, and weakness or heaviness of legs. Contact your doctor immediately if you experience fever and chills, hoarseness, swelling of face, mouth, hands or feet, sudden trouble with swallowing or breathing, stomach pain, itching or yellow eyes or skin.

Even so, these are probably the safest of the blood pressure drugs on offer.

Beta blockers

These drugs counter our normal stress response by preventing the heart from reacting to stress. They do this by reducing blood pressure. Beta blockers can sometimes help people with congestive heart failure by reducing tachycardia – that is, rapid heartbeats. They slow the heart rate. But there are major concerns about this class of drugs, especially one of the most commonly prescribed, atenolol.

Side effects Slowing the heart rate with beta blockers in people with hypertension is associated with an increased risk of cardio-vascular events and death, according to a systematic review in 2008.[56] Generally, slowing the heart rate is consistent with benefit, not harm. This review, however, found the opposite. According to some experts, the problem may have been the drug given, not the effect of slowing the heart rate. Most people in this trial were on atenolol. Dr John Cockcroft of the Wales Heart Institute commented, 'Atenolol has been tried and found guilty, and yet around 40 per cent of prescriptions for beta blockers in the UK and in the US are still for atenolol.' The same concern may not relate to newer beta blockers but this is certainly one to avoid. 'The newer vasodilating beta blockers may well not have any of these detrimental effects. Because they are vasodilatory, they may well offset the slowing of heart rate by decreasing wave reflection from the periphery and, in the case of nebivolol, by releasing nitric oxide, an endogenous vasodilator with antiatherogenic activity,' he adds.

There are real concerns about these drugs for anything other that short-term use or for people who have had heart attacks that have resulted in erratic heartbeats due to damage to the heart's left ventricle – beta blockers can reduce the risk of sudden cardiac death in these cases. These drugs also deplete CoQ_{10}, but to a much lesser extent than statins.

The Physician's Desk Reference, which is the book American doctors refer to on drugs, warns of the dangers of long-term use:

Cardiac Failure. Sympathetic stimulation is a vital component of supporting circulatory function in congestive heart failure, and a beta blockade carries the potential hazard of further depressing myocardial contractility and of precipitating more severe failure.

Patients Without a History of Cardiac Failure. Continued depression of the myocardium with beta blocking agents over a period of time can, in some cases, lead to cardiac failure.

Adverse Reactions – Cardiovascular. Shortness of breath and bradycardia (heart rate below 60) have occurred in approximately 3 of 100 patients. Cold extremities, arterial insufficiency of the Raynaud type, palpitations, congestive heart failure, peripheral edema, or hypotension have been reported in 1 of 100 patients.

So, if you've had cardiac failure these drugs could make it worse. If you haven't, long-term use could induce it.

That's not the end of the side effects, however. There is a host of less severe ones, including a decreased sex drive, insomnia, fatigue, dizziness and nausea.

If you want to come off beta blockers, be aware that you mustn't go cold turkey: this could precipitate angina, high blood pressure or even a heart attack. It is better to wean yourself off them. The elderly, pregnant women and people with kidney or thyroid disease should be especially cautious about taking beta blockers, and use the lowest dose possible to get their blood pressure under control – or follow the non-drug options outlined later in this chapter.

Calcium-channel blockers

The relaxation and tension of muscle cells depends on the balance between calcium and magnesium inside and out. One highly effective way to reduce blood pressure is to eat more magnesium (see Chapter 13). But calcium-channel blockers, like all the other hypertension drugs, block just one element in a carefully balanced system – in this case, the cell's ability to take up calcium. This forces the muscles in the arteries to relax.

The action of these drugs, which include verapamil, diltiazem and nifedipine, is bad news. Cells need calcium even if depriving them of it does lower blood pressure. A study in a 1995 issue of *Circulation*, the journal of the American Heart Association, showed that patients on one of the calcium-channel blockers – nifedipine – were more likely to die. As the paper said, 'High doses of nifedipine were significantly associated with increased mortality,' adding, 'Other calcium antagonists may have similar adverse effects.'[37] Norvasc is a newer version of this drug.

Side effects These include potassium loss, elevated serum choles-terol, headaches, dizziness, nausea, oedema, hypotension and constipation. Calcium-channel blockers also appear to affect the liver and interfere with carbohydrate metabolism and may not be suitable for diabetics for this reason.

Blood-thinning drugs

If you have blood that is prone to clotting, the abnormal heart rhythm known as atrial fibrillation, or you've had a heart attack or ischaemic stroke (that is, one involving a clot), you are very likely to be prescribed blood-thinning drugs. They're also used in medical emergencies and may be given in the short term if you are having an operation.

A stroke is essentially an injury to brain cells resulting from a disruption to blood flow. There are two main types of stroke. The first type are ischaemic, while the second type results from bleeding in the brain.

Warfarin

Warfarin, sold as coumadin in the US, is usually prescribed follow-ing an ischaemic stroke. Unfortunately, warfarin increases the risk of having a haemorrhagic stroke.

The case of Israel's former prime minister, Ariel Sharon, may be a tragic illustration of this. On 18 December 2005, Sharon had a mild ischaemic stroke from which he regained consciousness. His doctors gave him blood thinners, to prevent the blood from clotting.

However, according to a report in the British newspaper the *Guardian*, 'Doctors in Israel have admitted making a mistake when treating Israeli prime minister Ariel Sharon with large doses of blood thinners.' One of the doctors was quoted as saying that the anti-coagulants may have caused the debilitating haemorrhagic stroke that put him in a coma.[58]

Warfarin is also given to those with atrial fibrillation, which worsens blood flow, because it can reduce the risk of an embolic stroke by thinning the blood. Warfarin works by interfering with the formation of vitamin K, the body's natural blood clotting agent, in the liver, and the dose is managed by frequent blood tests to measure the time taken for blood to clot. This is known as the INR or international normalised ratio.

A normal INR is between 0.8 and 1.2. If you are taking warfarin because you're at high risk of a stroke or heart attack, your dose will be managed to achieve an INR of between 2 and 3 in most cases to prevent your blood from clotting too much. It's a fine balance because under-clotting carries its own risks.

Heparin

This drug is very similar to warfarin but can only be administered by injection, whereas warfarin is usually taken orally. It works faster and is usually prescribed with warfarin. Then, as warfarin starts to work, the patient is weaned off it.

Aspirin

Aspirin has an antiplatelet effect: it inhibits the hormone-like substances, prostaglandins, that encourage blood platelets to stick to each other and form blood clots. There is no similar measure of effectiveness to determine dose. In women over the age of 65, approximately 100mg of aspirin has been shown to have a mild benefit in preventing stroke, but the overuse of aspirin causes thousands of deaths a year from gastrointestinal bleeding.

Don't use aspirin to prevent heart disease. Although aspirin has been prescribed to millions of people over the past 20 years the current evidence is that the benefits don't outweigh the risks. The British Heart Foundation no longer recommends it for prevention, following a number of major analyses which found that the benefit you were likely to get was more or less the same as your risk of having serious internal bleeding – one of the well-known side effects of aspirin. In both cases about 350–400 people had to be treated for one to benefit or to be harmed – not exactly good odds. One study, for example, followed 29,000 people over eight years taking either an enteric-coated aspirin or a placebo. There was no difference in cardiovascular events or deaths, but a small increase in risk of hospital admission for a major haemorrhage (internal bleeding).[59]

The first paper was a little hesitant saying that 'aspirin is of uncertain net value as the reduction in occlusive events i.e. blocked arteries'.[60] The second didn't beat about the bush. Its title said it all: 'Don't use aspirin for primary prevention of cardiovascular disease'.[61] And the third was just as clear: 'Use of aspirin in primary prevention of cardiovascular disease ... is not supported by the current evidence'.[62] The latest concludes: 'The current totality of evidence provides only modest support for a benefit of aspirin in patients without clinical cardiovascular disease, which is offset by its risk. For every 1,000 subjects treated with aspirin over a 5-year period, aspirin would prevent 2.9 major cardiovascular events and cause 2.8 major bleeds.'[63]

I think you'll agree that this is pretty unambiguous. But not only was the British Heart Foundation's reversal of a recommendation they had been pushing for years announced in the equivalent of a whisper but also GPs have effectively ignored the whole thing. The prescribing of low-dose aspirin in England before those papers came out was around 32 million per year; the following year it was 31 million.

What if you've got heart disease and are at increased risk of a blood clot? The picture here is not so clear. A recent study followed 39,500 people over a three-year period who had had cardiovascular disease and either stayed on or discontinued aspirin. There was no difference in risk of dying, but those who stopped aspirin had a slight increased risk of a non-fatal heart attack with four more heart attacks per 1,000 people per year. Strangely, this study didn't report on the number of incidents of internal bleeding in those staying on aspirin, although they state that 'recorded safety concerns were the second most common reason for discontinuation in this study'.[64] Studies are now underway to evaluate benefit versus risk in those with cardio-vascular disease.

Blood-thinning drugs: the side effects

The major side effect of the blood-thinning drugs is excessive bleeding, such as eye and brain haemorrhages, blood in the urine, and bleeding gums. Warfarin can also cause hypersensitivity, hair loss, rashes, diarrhoea, 'purple toes', liver dysfunction, nausea and vomiting.[65] Aspirin causes gastrointestinal bleeding, as we've seen, and should be avoided if you have gut problems, a history of haemorrhagic stroke, bleeding ulcers, haemorrhoids, bleeding into the eyes or diabetes. While anticoagulants help prevent thrombotic and embolic strokes, the risk of a stroke-induced haemorrhage is actually higher for those taking warfarin and aspirin. Note that you should never take warfarin and aspirin at the same time.

A note on natural blood-thinners

A number of supplements that are highly beneficial for the heart also thin the blood. Garlic, gingko and fish oil are generally not recommended if you're taking blood-thinning drugs: there have been some isolated reports of bleeding on gingko and long-term aspirin therapy. It is also wise to limit your intake of vitamin E to no more than 300mg if you're on one of these drugs.

However, it has to be said that you can't have it both ways. If these nutrients do substantially thin the blood, and they do, they are obviously preferable to blood-thinning drugs. So, perhaps the caution should read: 'Do not take warfarin or aspirin if you are supplementing large or combined amounts of omega-3 fish oils, vitamin E, gingko biloba and garlic.' But since the effect of these nutrients is less imme-diate and less quantifiable, they shouldn't be used in the short term after a medical crisis. They could be used to reduce the need for anticoagulant drugs once your condition and your INR are stable

– although if you are on warfarin, you should stick to food sources of these nutrients, not concentrated daily supplements.

It's best to discuss all this with your doctor to ensure that your INR is monitored as you increase the nutrients, so that he or she can reduce the drugs accordingly.

PART 2

TEN KEYS FOR PREVENTING AND REVERSING HEART DISEASE

Now you know what heart disease is all about, and how you measure risk, what are the real underlying causes and what can you do to reverse your risk? In this part you'll discover what's really driving heart disease and what to do about it. Heart disease is not caused by a lack of drugs, and its treatment should not be primarily based on this. It is caused, as you'll see, by our modern-day diet, its concomitant lack of nutrients, and a stressful lifestyle devoid of exercise. Also, the level of nutrients you need to reverse risk is quite different from that needed to maintain basic health. In this part you'll discover the nutrients that work better than drugs.

CHAPTER 7

Why You Need Omega-3 Fats and Vitamin D

One of the biggest mistakes made in nutrition has been the tyranny against fats. It has fuelled fat phobia and contributed to a big decrease in consumption of essential fats from oily fish such as salmon, mackerel and sardines. Despite eating less fat, the number of obese people has gone through the roof, largely due to eating more carbs which, as you'll see in the next chapter, is another big driver of heart disease.

The enigma of the Eskimos

Back in 1974, Dr Hugh Sinclair, a medical scientist from Oxford University, was perplexed by the enigma of the Inuit people living in the Arctic Circle. Despite an incredibly high-fat and -cholesterol diet, they had virtually no heart disease. He went to investigate and came back to England armed with enough seal meat, fish, crustaceans and molluscs to live off for 100 days. During that time his blood became less thick, his triglyceride (blood fat) level dropped and his HDL levels, the 'good cholesterol', increased.[1] He had found the elixir that had protected the Inuit: a diet of foods exceptionally rich in the essential fatty acid EPA.

Thanks to the unusual diet of the late Sir Hugh (subsequently knighted for his contribution to moving medicine forward), a number of studies in the 1980s further investigated the health benefits of EPA in relation to the health of the heart and arteries. It became increasingly clear that a high intake of oily fish was remarkably protective.

The Japanese lifestyle is an interesting example. Despite above average levels of drinking and smoking, the Japanese have a history of longevity unparalleled by other industrialised countries. Like the Inuit, one dietary difference is a high fish intake. In 1980 an analysis of blood levels of EPA among the Japanese population did indeed show much higher levels of EPA than those found in British or American populations, and especially among fish-eating, rather than farming, communities.[2] As a consequence, they may live longer and suffer less heart disease.[3] (There is another critical nutrient in oily fish, vitamin D, which is also associated with reducing risk of heart disease, and I'll discuss this in detail later in this chapter.)

Foods rich in omega-3

As we saw in Chapter 4, reducing overall fat intake results in a reduction in heart disease risk only if you replace some of the saturated fat, largely from animal products, with polyunsaturated fats – and these come from fish, raw nuts and seeds.

Polyunsaturated fat, unlike saturated fat (which can only be used for fuel or padding), contains essential omega-3 and 6 fats that have all sorts of health benefits. The typical Western diet is much more deficient in omega-3 fats, from which the body makes anti-inflammatory prostaglandins. These lower cholesterol and triglycerides, decrease blood pressure, prevent blood clotting and raise HDLs. No drug has that kind of all-round heart-friendly action, without side effects (although you have to be careful if you are on blood-thinning drugs, because omega-3s do a similar thing, see page 74).

As you can see in the illustration on page 71, certain seeds, notably those that grow in a cold climate, are a rich, root source of omega-3s, called alpha-linolenic acid (ALA). The best food sources are chia seeds, grown in Central America at altitude, flax seeds and also walnuts. Hemp and pumpkin seeds, especially if from a colder

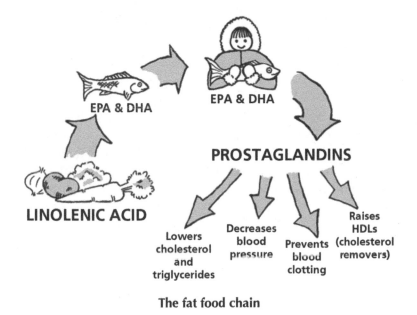

The fat food chain

climate, are quite good sources too. About 5 per cent of ALA is converted into EPA, which is the most potent anti-inflammatory form of omega-3.

Eating a tablespoonful of chia or flax seeds or a small handful of walnuts a day has some cardiovascular benefit, plus other benefits – all are high in protein, vitamins and minerals. Chia seeds are the best all-rounder. They are exceptionally high in soluble fibre, which also helps clear excess cholesterol and stabilises blood sugar levels. They also taste much nicer than flax.

This vegetarian source of omega-3 is, however, probably not enough on its own to have a big impact but they do help reduce risk.

In the Nurses' Health Study, involving 76,763 nurses aged between 30 and 55 years old who were monitored for 18 years, the greater their intake of ALA the less was their risk of sudden cardiac death (but not other types of fatal CHD such as heart attacks and strokes). Those with the highest intake, around 1.16g each day, cut their risk of cardiac death by a third.[4]

Another study gave people margarine either containing 1.9g of ALA, or nothing. Among the women in this study, the ALA group was associated with a 27 per cent reduction in major cardiovascular events when compared to those who had the plain margarine.[5]

If you have a tablespoon of, for example, chia seeds you get 2.2g of ALA, while two dessertspoons is 2.9g. It may be that higher levels of ALA are more effective, especially for women. There is some evidence that women make better use of dietary ALA than men.

Oily fish (that is cold-water fish that eat other fish) are, however, a very rich source of the more potent form of omega-3, called eicosapentaenoic acid or EPA for short. In head-to-head trials, EPA does work much better than vegetarian sources of ALA.[6] Most trials give something like 1g of EPA, which is the kind of level you would find in two high-potency fish oil capsules or two servings of oily fish, such as mackerel.

The evidence for omega-3 is substantial

Increasing your intake of omega-3 fish oils, both by eating fish and by supplementing fish oils, is a must for anyone with cardiovascular risk. A 2004 review of ten randomised controlled trials showed that fish oils decrease triglycerides by an average of 29 per cent, lower cholesterol by 12 per cent, lower the bad LDL cholesterol by 32 per cent and increase HDL by 10 per cent.[7] They also offer anti-inflammatory benefits, which is at the heart of arterial disease.[8] In a trial in Sheffield with 100 cardiac patients, virtually everyone achieved normal triglycerides and much-reduced angina medication after a year on EPA.[9]

Basically, they are a lot more effective than statins and have a range of other beneficial effects. The trouble is you can't patent them so they are not particularly profitable and therefore not promoted in the same way.

A long-term study comparing the effects of giving patients with heart failure cholesterol-lowering statin drugs or omega-3 fish oils has shown that the omega-3 fats cut the risk of death or hospitalisation, compared to placebo, while the statins don't. Those taking 1g a day of omega-3 fats cut their risk of mortality by 9 per cent and risk of admission to hospital by 8 per cent compared to placebo. Those taking statins had no reduction in risk.[10]

Another study gave over 18,000 Japanese people with high cholesterol (above 6.5mmol/l) either high-dose fish oils (1.8g of EPA) with statins, or just statins. After six years those on the EPA had reduced the risk of a major coronary event by 19 per cent in those who had cardiovascular disease.[11] There were also fewer non-fatal coronary events and angina problems in those who did have heart disease at the start of the study. (Bear in mind that people in Japan have a much higher intake of omega-3 to start with so an even greater benefit would be expected in British people.)

The strongest evidence for the effectiveness of omega-3s, however, lies in their ability to reduce the risk of a heart attack if you've already had one. Eating only one serving of oily fish a week cuts your likelihood of having another heart attack by a third. As a study published in 1999 showed, supplementing omega-3 fish oils also cuts your risk of dying from cardiovascular disease by 21 per cent.[12] In the *British Medical Journal* in 2004, a review of the many studies that consistently show benefit from omega-3-rich fish oils concludes: 'Omega-3 fatty acids from fish and fish oils can protect against coronary heart disease. There is evidence to support the use of fish or fish oil supplements after myocardial infarction.'[13]

However, it's not all plain sailing for omega-3s vis-à-vis heart health. A review in the *British Medical Journal* published in 2006 looked at 12 studies (9 showing a benefit, 1 no effect and 2 a very small negative effect), and didn't find a clear reduction in mortality.[14] So don't put all your fish in one basket.

Overall, the evidence is certainly strong enough for the UK's National Institute for Health and Clinical Excellence (NICE) to recommend all doctors prescribe 1g of fish oil a day for six months to patients who have had a heart attack (after this time, the budget runs out!).

A word of caution if you are on blood thinners

As we've seen, fish oils also help to thin the blood, so if you're already on blood-thinning medication such as warfarin or aspirin you should consult your doctor before taking them so that he or she can closely monitor your international normalised ratio or INR – that is, how well your blood coagulates.[15] (See page 65 for a fuller discussion of this issue.) Given the broad benefits of omega-3 fish oils, and the limited benefit and side effects of aspirin, omega-3s would be a better choice provided you are being appropriately monitored.

The best fish to eat

Although it may not be environmentally correct, with declining levels of fish in the sea, and an increasing population, the optimal intake of oily/carnivorous fish is three to five servings a week. NICE, which advises NHS policy, recommends all heart attack patients eat two to four portions of oily fish (herring, sardines, mackerel, salmon, tuna and trout) a week.

In our 100% Health Survey, we gathered information on health and diet from 55,000 people, and found that a person's chances of being in optimal health goes up by a third for those consuming three or more servings of oily fish a week, compared to two a week. A portion is defined as 140g (5oz), which is a small can of fish or a small fillet of fresh fish, from which one should derive at least 7g of omega-3 essential fats over a week.

Not all oily fish are equal

Have a look at the chart on page 75 and you will see that the level of omega-3s is a fraction in canned tuna compared to fresh. This is probably because the oil may be squeezed out, and may be sold to the supplement industry, leaving a drier meat disguised as such by putting the tuna in another oil. In the US you can buy tuna in its own oil. It tastes completely different and much better. So don't rely on canned tuna to provide your omega-3 quota, always try to use fresh fish. Another problem with oily fish is the potential for mercury contamination, particularly in very large fish such as tuna. This is particularly relevant for pregnant women, because mercury is a neurotoxin and can induce birth defects. I would recommend tuna no more than once a fortnight during pregnancy and once a week or fortnight otherwise. The same advice applies to marlin or swordfish. The best all-rounders are probably wild salmon and mackerel. The level of omega-3 in farmed salmon is largely going to depend upon what they are fed.

Fish Source FSA 2004	Omega-3 g/100g	EPA g/100g	Mercury mg/kg	Omega-3/mercury ratio
Canned tuna	0.37	0.23	0.19	1.95
Trout	1.15	0.25	0.06	19.17
Herring	1.31	0.90	0.04	32.75
Fresh tuna	1.50	0.09	0.40	3.75
Canned/smoked salmon	1.54	0.47	0.04	38.50
Canned sardines	1.57	0.47	0.04	39.25
Fresh mackerel	1.93	0.65	0.05	38.60
Fresh salmon	2.70	0.69	0.05	54.00
Swordfish	2?	0.13	1.40	1.43?
Marlin	2?		1.10	1.83?

The omega-3 and mercury content of fish

Oily fish possesses other health benefits unrelated to its omega-3 levels, being very high in protein, vitamin E and selenium, so I would always advise eating your three portions a week (just don't count canned tuna), but I also suggest supplementing as well, especially on those days that you don't eat fish.

The vitamin D factor

The single most important source of vitamin D is oily fish, although most is made in your skin in the presence of sunlight. If you live in Northern Europe the chances are very high that you do not get enough vitamin D. We need about 20 minutes of sun exposure a day, with as much skin exposed as possible, to synthesise vitamin D.

In the spirit of Hugh Sinclair's investigation of the Inuit, Dr David Grimes, from the Department of Medicine and Biochemistry at Blackburn Royal Infirmary in the north-west of England, wondered why heart disease incidence varied across the UK, and also why heart attacks were much more common in the winter months. By analysing data from across the UK and also from around the world, he showed that cholesterol levels also go up the further you live from the equator and the less time you spend outdoors. Exposure to sunlight converts cholesterol in the skin into health-promoting vitamin D.[16] One real possibility is that, in the absence of enough direct sunlight, we accumulate cholesterol.

While it has long been known that the further south you go the less the risk of heart disease, this was assumed to be due to dietary differences, but Grimes and others have shown that sun exposure through the seasons directly changes cholesterol levels. Since Grimes's research in the 1990s, there have been plenty of studies showing that the lower your vitamin D level the greater your risk of heart disease.

According to Dr James O'Keefe of the Mid America Heart Institute in Kansas City, 'Vitamin D deficiency is an unrecognised, emerging cardiovascular risk factor, which should be screened for and treated.'[17] In 2011, he reported that testing the vitamin D levels of 239 patients arriving in hospital with a heart attack revealed that 96 per cent had 'abnormally low' levels.[18]

It appears that your vitamin D level should not be below 75 nmol/l, and if your level is below 35 nmol/l your risk is certainly going to be higher.[19] Your doctor can easily test this for you or you can do it yourself privately (see Resources). An ideal vitamin D level for overall health (it also protects bones, strengthens your immune system and reduces the risk of cancer) is a blood level above 100 nmol/l.

It appears that the problem can start very early in life. Dr Michael Burch, of Great Ormond Street Hospital, London, has estimated that 25 per cent of the cases of babies with heart failure are due to vitamin D deficiency. He reports on a few cases where babies scheduled for a transplant recovered rapidly when supplemented with vitamin D.[20]

Exactly how vitamin D protects the heart is not yet clear, but one way is probably by keeping the endothelium (the very fine lining of blood vessels) flexible, making you less likely to suffer with high blood pressure. Researchers checked the vitamin D levels of over 500 healthy staff at Emory University in Georgia and found that those with a deficiency had vascular dysfunction comparable to those with diabetes or hypertension.[21]

We will have to wait for trials giving vitamin D to find out if supplementation is protective for all, or just those with very low levels. It is quite likely that a lack of vitamin D doesn't cause heart disease, but allows cholesterol to accumulate and blood pressure to rise, thus making existing risk factors worse. This may also be why drug trials tend to be less effective in areas with low sun exposure. (See Chapter 18 for more on vitamin D and what to do if you have high blood pressure.)

Summary

Here's what to do:

Omega-3s

- Fish oils contain two kinds of omega-3s: EPA and DHA. It's the EPA that particularly seems to reduce the risk of heart attacks and strokes. A serving of oily fish, such as a piece of organic salmon, can provide around 3g of omega-3 fats. Of this perhaps a quarter, 800mg, is EPA. You should aim for around 400mg of EPA a day, minimum. That's either two high-potency omega-3 fish oil capsules a day, or half a serving of an omega-3-rich fish such as sardines, herring or mackerel. Having three servings of fish each week and an omega-3 fish oil capsule providing around 200mg of EPA a day is a good place to start.

- If you already have cardiovascular disease, you might want to double this by supplementing 400mg of EPA a day, and eating oily fish at least three times a week. In practical terms this means having one or two high-potency omega-3-rich fish oil capsules every day, plus eating oily fish.
- In any event, eat oily fish at least three times a week. It is a good source of both omega-3 and vitamin D.

Vitamin D

- Get your vitamin D level checked and aim to get it above 75nmol/l and ideally above 100nmol/l.
- Take a high-potency multivitamin providing 15mcg of vitamin D. In the winter months add 25–50mcg of vitamin as 1 or 2 drops of a high-potency vitamin D oil if you live in Northern Europe.
- Get out in the sunlight as much as you can.

Chapter 22 helps you build your own supplement programme.

CHAPTER 8

The Sugar Factor and Why You Need to Keep Your Insulin Down

The simplest and fastest way to reduce your risk of heart disease and lower almost every indicator of risk is to eat a low-GL (glycemic load) diet – in other words avoid sugars and refined carbohydrates and always eat protein with carbohydrate. Foods such as sugar and refined foods have a high 'glycemic load' which means that they raise your blood glucose level drastically followed by a rapid drop. Fluctuations in blood sugar levels lead to excess weight and a feeling of exhaustion. Plus, the high levels of insulin that have to be released to process the sugar have many bad effects on the body. As we've already seen, a low-GL diet is an effective way of controlling high cholesterol levels, for example. This means eating a bit less carbohydrate, and consciously choosing those that release their sugar content slowly, plus eating a bit more protein. By combining protein with carbohydrate in a meal (such as oats with ground seeds, or brown rice with fish, or eggs with oatcakes), you further lower the speed of glucose release into the blood, thus lowering your 'glycemic load'.

Researchers at the Harvard School of Public Health carried out a massive survey of the dietary habits and health risks of 82,802 women during 20 years of follow up. Their study showed that a high-GL diet almost doubles (95 per cent) the risk of heart disease compared to a low-GL diet.[22] They also found that diets that provide more protein from vegetable sources lower cardiovascular risk. This confirms an earlier study involving 75,000 nurses in which those with a high-GL diet doubled their risk of heart disease.[23]

When you eat too much carbohydrate on a regular basis, especially sweet foods or those made with refined carbohydrates, such as white flour, white rice or sugar, three things happen that are very bad news for your cardiovascular system:

1   You get too many blood sugar peaks, where glucose can start to damage the arteries, the kidneys and cholesterol particles in the arteries via a process called glycosylation. Damaged cholesterol leads to raised LDL cholesterol and the immune system attacking cells and producing foam cells, engorged with cholesterol. Your kidney function goes downhill, which raises blood pressure. The arteries can't function properly leading to less effective reception for insulin.

2   You start to become insulin insensitive, which means you release even more insulin. This, in turn, raises water and the sodium content in the blood, which raises your blood pressure. Insulin also stops you breaking down fat, so your cholesterol and triglyceride levels start to rise.

3   You also get rebound blood sugar lows, which trigger the release of adrenal hormones, increasing your stress level and your blood pressure, and your body channels energy into 'fight or flight' and away from healing, for example, your damaged arteries. (You'll find more on this in Chapter 9.)

The glycemic index and glycemic load

You may have heard of the glycemic index. This is slightly different from the glycemic load. The glycemic index is a *qualitative* measure that tells you whether the kind of carbohydrate in the food converts rapidly or slowly into glucose. The glycemic load of a food takes the *quantity* and the *quality* into account – it is literally the quantity of carbs in the serving of a food multiplied by the quality of its carbohydrate, i.e. its glycemic index. The glycemic load is a more accurate and practical way to achieve blood sugar control.

Proof that a low-GL diet lowers cholesterol and risk

Many studies show that low-GL diets have immediate and long-term benefits for your health, including lowering total cholesterol, raising 'good' HDL cholesterol, stabilising blood glucose levels and improving insulin sensitivity, and reducing cardiovascular disease risk. Here are some examples:

A low-GL diet improves cardiovascular health – the evidence

- Two groups of overweight or obese people followed either a low-GL diet or a low-fat, low-calorie diet for two years. Those on the low-GL diet had greater improvements in insulin resistance (blood sugar control), triglycerides (fat circulating in the blood), inflammation and blood pressure compared with those on the conventional low-fat, low-calorie diet. The researchers concluded that a reduction in glycemic load may aid in the prevention or treatment of obesity, cardiovascular disease, and diabetes mellitus.[24]
- One group of people followed a low-GL diet while another group followed a conventional low-fat, low-calorie diet (Canada's Food Guide to Healthy Eating). After six months those following the low-GL diet lost more weight; they also had greater improvements in HDL cholesterol, triglycerides and fasting glucose compared to those on the conventional low-fat, low-calorie diet. These health gains were sustained or improved upon after 12 months. The researchers concluded that 'implementation of a low-GL diet is associated with substantial and sustained improvements in abdominal obesity, cholesterol and blood sugar control'. [25]
- A study was published in the *Lancet* in 2004 in which two groups of mice were fed either a low-GL diet or a high-GL diet and their health compared. Besides being leaner, the low-GL group had better blood sugar control and lower blood fats.[26]

- A study of 574 adults in Massachusetts between 1994 and 1997 found that higher total carbohydrate intake, percentage of calories from carbohydrate and glycemic index/glycemic load were related to lower levels of beneficial HDL cholesterol and higher blood triglyceride levels. These results show an unfavourable effect of increased intake of highly processed carbohydrate on fat profile, increasing cardiovascular risk.[27]

- Participants in this study were assigned to either a low-fat diet or one of two kinds of Mediterranean diet. Those in the Mediterranean diet groups received nutritional education plus either free virgin olive oil (1 litre/1¾ pints per week) or free nuts (30g/1oz per day). Changes were evaluated after three months. Compared with the low-fat diet, the Mediterranean diet produced more beneficial changes in blood sugar levels, blood pressure and good HDL cholesterol. The Mediterranean diet with olive oil also reduced levels of the dangerous C-reactive protein, associated with heart disease. These results show that a Mediterranean-style diet, which promotes low-GL carbohydrates and increased monounsaturated fat intake, is more beneficial than a low-fat diet.[28]

- Twelve men with type-2 diabetes followed a low-GL or high-GL diet for four weeks. Blood sugar levels after a meal were significantly lower in people following the low-GL diet than those in the high-GL diet. Insulin levels and 'bad' LDL cholesterol were also lower in the low-GL group.[29]

- Another study, this time from Italy, called the EPICOR trial, which involved more than 47,000 people, compared diet with cardiovascular risk over almost eight years. Those women in the top quarter of glycemic load (GL) diets – that is, eating the most carbs in the form of fast-releasing sugar and refined foods – had double the risk of coronary heart disease than those in the lowest quarter. This study didn't find the same association with men.[30] However, a study from Holland found that men with a higher GL diet had a 17 per cent increased risk of coronary heart disease with a less significant 9 per cent increase in women.[31]

- A study published in the *Archives of Internal Medicine* shows excellent results. Headed by Professor David Jenkins, the study gave two groups of people a reduced-calorie diet: one with a low amount of carbohydrates (with low-glycemic index ratings) and high protein and fat, but from vegetable sources; the other with higher carbohydrates, and lower fat and protein. Both groups lost almost 4kg (9lb) in the four weeks, but those on the low-carb diet had greater reductions in their total cholesterol and LDL cholesterol levels.[32]

Even back in 2007 a meta-analysis of weight-loss studies concluded that: 'Overweight or obese people lost more weight on a low-Glycemic diet and had more improvement in lipid [that is, cholesterol and triglyceride] profiles than those receiving conventional [low-fat] diets.'[33] Other benefits were a greater loss in body fat, a reduction in 'bad' LDL cholesterol and an increase in 'good' HDL cholesterol. I sincerely hope that in the next five years the recommendation to eat a low-fat diet to lose weight or reduce your risk of cardiovascular disease will become a thing of the past, replaced by the recommendation to eat low-GL.

You may remember that in Chapter 1 I explained about the trial where a group of GPs put 21 patients fitting the category of metabolic syndrome, with high risk of heart disease and diabetes, on my low-GL diet as part of our Zest4Life programme. In just 12 weeks triglycerides, cholesterol and LDL cholesterol all dropped, while 'good' HDL cholesterol increased. Total cholesterol dropped by 13 per cent, from 5.3mmol/l to 4.6mmol, while the cholesterol to HDL ratio dropped by 9 per cent, from 4.1 to 3.7. Blood pressure also reduced. You can see the full results on pages 17–18. This scale of improvement is rarely seen on drug regimes. All of this is consistent with a reduced risk of heart disease, as well as other diseases.

A low-GL diet plus supplements works best

I should remind you that the above successful results were achieved in a mere 12 weeks, and without the use of any supplements. Normally,

I would recommend someone to supplement omega-3 fish oils, a high-strength multivitamin and mineral, plus niacin, for reasons that will become clear.

Case Study: Andrew

Andrew, from Dublin, had a cholesterol level of 8.8 mmol/l. He was put on statins and, six months later, his cholesterol was 8.7. The lack of response, plus unpleasant side effects, led him to stop. He described himself as very stressed, and tired. He had five coffees a day to keep himself going and found it hard to relax in the evening and would have a couple of drinks. He was also gaining weight and not sleeping well.

He heard me on television asking for a volunteer with high cholesterol for a three-week experiment and rang up the station. I put him on my low-GL diet and recommended certain supplements. Three weeks later we met at the TV station for the 'reveal'. He had lost 4.5kg (10lb), his energy levels were great, he no longer felt stressed and he was sleeping much better. We then tested his cholesterol and it had dropped to a healthy 4.9!

Keeping your blood sugar level even not only helps you to lose weight but gives you more energy and makes you less stressed. That's because blood sugar peaks and troughs trigger adrenal hormones. These make you more likely to react stressfully, and also promote the body's equivalent of stress, which is called inflammation. Inflammation, in turn, leads to heart disease.

The rapid transformation in Andrew might sound amazing, but I hear it all the time. Like the lady I met recently who went to her doctor for a check-up and was told that she had high blood pressure and cholesterol and would need to take cholesterol-lowering statins and blood pressure drugs. She didn't want to take drugs for the rest of her life.

'My doctor told me that if it wasn't reduced within about eight weeks, I would have to go on statins and blood-pressure tablets. After going to the nurse for six weeks, nothing was happening and I decided to take control and to go on a diet. So I joined Zest4Life. Within ten weeks I lost 26 lbs [11.8kg (1 stone 12lb)]. I returned to the doctor who tested my blood pressure and sent me for a cholesterol test, both of which were lowered, and the result is that I do not need to go on the statins!'

Eating a low-GL diet also lowers your blood pressure

A low-GL diet is also an excellent way to lower blood pressure (BP), which is one of the top risk factors for heart disease and stroke. Even so, millions of people are given drugs, as we saw in Chapter 6. You may be prescribed a combination of two different types in one, with the promise of even more effective lowering. The trouble is that some types of drug make you pee more, and the more you pee the more minerals you lose, including potassium and magnesium, which actually lower blood pressure.

By following a low-GL diet you avoid blood sugar dips, which trigger blood pressure-raising adrenal hormones, but also the less insulin you make the less sodium and water accumulate in the blood. If your blood sugar level isn't too high the body won't need to dilute it with water. You may remember David from the Introduction. Here is more of his story:

Case Study: David
David had spent ten years trying to sort out his hypertension using drugs, with limited benefits, before he discovered that the low-GL diet could do it in six months.

In 1996, at the age of 44, David was diagnosed with high blood pressure and told that he would have to take beta blockers, which stop the heart from being stimulated by adrenalin, for the rest of his life.

'They [the beta blockers] made it almost impossible for me to exercise. Running felt as if I was carrying a couple of sacks of potatoes.'

So he decided to find another way.

'I had a good diet and I exercised, so I wanted to find out why I was having this problem. I bought a blood pressure meter and I started to do my own research.'

With regular monitoring, he discovered that his blood pressure was very unstable.

'It would be low for a while after I took the drug, but then it would rise out of control. The doctors call it "resistive hypertension".'

He showed his results to a cardiology lecturer who agreed to help, and he ran a lot of tests, which eventually showed David that he had rather high levels of a hormone called aldosterone. The doctor put him on an alpha-blocker instead, which allowed him to start exercising regularly again. But things still weren't right, so David was passed on to a professor at a large hospital in London.

'He was shocked that my blood pressure was so high and he struggled to treat me for a year, but despite more tests and scans we got nowhere. Eventually, we found a high-potassium diet seemed to help. So I went on a diuretic that conserved potassium and two other drugs which brought my blood pressure down, and it stayed down.'

But the idea of staying on those drugs indefinitely didn't appeal. So ten years after he'd started on his quest, David decided to try out my low-GL diet. The results were rapid and impressive.

'Within about three weeks I started feeling giddy, and my monitor showed my blood pressure had dropped right down, so I halved my medication. But two weeks later the same thing happened and I had to come off my medication completely!'

Two months later, David took his blood pressure figures to the professor.

'He was astonished and highly delighted. Then I broke the news to him that those figures had been achieved without any medication at all! The initial look of horror on his face changed to total fascination when I explained it was all the result of the low-GL diet and that a further benefit was that my cholesterol had dropped from 5.7 to 4.6.'

Three years later David is still eating low-GL and not taking any tablets. Not everyone achieves a result as good as this, but many are able to come off their pills. It has to be a better way.

Test yourself to see how much you could benefit

Although everyone can benefit from following a low-GL diet, just how important this factor is for you is easily determined by a simple measure called 'glycosylated haemoglobin'. A glycosylated haemoglobin test is available through doctors or a home-test kit (called a GL Check) may be used. It is a very good indicator of your risk of heart disease (and the best single indicator of diabetes risk, better than the standard blood glucose test).[34] More and more experts are recommending that it becomes part of screening for cardiovascular risk, especially in those people with blood sugar problems or abdominal weight gain.[35]

Here's how you do it:

1   You buy the kit (see Resources), which contains a device that pricks your finger (it doesn't hurt).

2   Put the lancet on your finger or thumb, press the purple part of the lancet down to pierce your skin. Massage your finger or thumb until there are large droplets of blood.

3   Hold your finger or thumb directly over the orange tube to drop the blood in. Keep massaging to produce a few droplets of blood until it reaches the orange line.

4   Immediately, place the orange tube inside the larger container tube. Put this and the used lancets in the prepaid envelope provided and return to the laboratory the same day.

5   They will send you a result that looks like this:

Personal Details

Name:	Mr Example Results	Gender:	Male
DOB:	18 November 1978	Age:	32
Weight:	85kg	Height:	1.82metres

Body Mass Index (BMI) score: 25.6

Glycosylated haemoglobin level: 6.5%   Normal range <5.5%

GLCheck result

Your overall GL Check score is DARK AMBER

Optimum 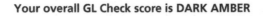 High

Glycosylated haemoglobin (HbA1c) test results

As you look at the results chart, you want to be in the white area (with a GL Check score below 5.5 per cent), not in the black (above 7 per cent). If you have a score in the dark grey range (6.1–6.9 per cent), you are at risk of developing diabetes or heart disease, and you probably already have a degree of insulin resistance and metabolic syndrome. If you are in the light grey range (5.5–6 per cent) you are out of danger, with mild dysglycemia, but with room for improvement in relation to your diet. (Note: your actual lab results will be in colour, ascending in risk from green through amber to red.)

If you score between 6 and 6.5 per cent, you've increased your risk of heart disease by more than a quarter and quadrupled your risk of diabetes. If you score above 6.5 per cent you have double the risk of cardiovascular disease and 16 times the risk of diabetes.[36] A score above 7 per cent is indicative of diabetes, or certainly pre-diabetes with a concomitant high risk of heart disease.

Conversely, decreasing your score by 1 per cent gives you a 16 per cent decreased risk of heart failure and a 43 per cent reduced risk of amputation or death caused by peripheral vascular disease.

Other studies have shown that, on its own, the glycosylated haemoglobin test is a highly sensitive test for either diagnosing or predicting the development of diabetes[37] and for predicting cardiovascular disease.[38] For example, a recent Japanese study of 7,832 patients with slightly high cholesterol but no cardiovascular disease found that, five years later, those who had an HbA1c score of over 6.5 per cent, compared to those below 6 per cent, had increased their risk of having developed cardiovascular disease by 2.4 times.[39]

If your score is high (above 5.5 per cent) it is imperative that you follow a low-GL diet – my Heart-friendly Diet – but in truth it is worth doing anyway because it is simply the best healthy diet going.

The power of vegetable protein and soluble fibres

One of the ways of lowering the glycemic load of your diet is to increase your intake of protein. The best kind of protein is vegetable protein, from beans, lentils, nuts and seeds, because these are also high in another natural cholesterol-lowering agent: plant sterols. You might have heard of these plant sterols because they are added to some 'cholesterol-lowering' margarines. They are also found richly in soya, which is why soya products often say 'helps lower your cholesterol'. They do.

If you eat protein *with* carbohydrate this further helps to slow the release of sugars in the food, since protein takes longer to digest than carbs.

Another way to lower the GL of a meal is to include foods rich in soluble fibres. These absorb more water and become a bit 'glooky' when soaked or cooked with water. Oats are a superb source of these fibres, and that's why porridge looks like it does. These soluble fibres also help eliminate excess cholesterol.

My low-GL diet is naturally rich in these two cholesterol-lowering compounds: plant sterols (found in beans, nuts and seeds), and soluble fibres (found in oats, barley, aubergines and okra). Putting all these factors together is especially effective.

Professor David Jenkins, from the University of Toronto, put 34 patients with high cholesterol on several different dietary combinations for a month. Some were on a low-fat diet, another group had a low-fat diet plus statins, and a third group was given lots of plant sterols and soluble fibres.[40]

This group ate the equivalent of 2.5g of plant sterols per day from the following foods:

50g (1¾oz) of soya (a glass of soya milk, or a small serving of tofu, or a small soya burger) and 35g (1¼oz) of almonds (a small handful of almonds); plus 25g (1oz) of soluble fibres from oats and vegetables (the equivalent of five oatcakes, plus a bowl of oats and three servings of vegetables).

Both statins and the plant sterol–soluble fibre diet significantly lowered LDL cholesterol to the same degree, but nine of the volunteers (26 per cent) achieved their lowest LDL cholesterol while on the plant sterol–soluble fibre diet, not the statins.

The four principles of low-GL eating

Foods are measured in GLs, which is literally the effect the food has on your blood sugar levels. In Part 4 I'll be giving you full details and in Appendix I will give you a list of foods with their GL values. If you need to lose weight, you will get the best results if you eat and drink no more than 45GLs in carbohydrate a day, spread out evenly throughout the day and always eaten with protein foods. This is just about the lowest you can go without ever feeling hungry. (If you are more than 1.8m (6ft) tall and you exercise a lot you'll need more. See Appendix 2 for a chart showing the GLs you'll need depending on your height and exercise level.) If you don't need to lose weight you can increase your carbs to 65GLs a day for general cardiovascular health. To achieve this there are only four principles you need to adhere to:

1 Eat 45GLs a day (or 65GLs for the 'maintenance' diet) You'll be learning exactly what the GL of a food is. Some foods have such a high-GL score that you would only be able to eat the smallest amount of them; for example, a whole 300g (10½oz) punnet of strawberries is 5GLs but so are just 10 raisins!

2 Graze rather than gorge Eat less food, more often. Divide the GLs throughout the day as follows:

10GLs for breakfast
5GLs for a mid-morning snack
10GLs for lunch
5GLs for a mid-afternoon snack
10GLs for dinner
5GLs for drinks or desserts

You'll soon know exactly what a 5GL snack or a 10GL main meal means.

3 Eat fewer carbs, but more protein You can achieve a low-GL diet in one of two ways: the first is by eating no, or less, carbohydrate, since only carbohydrates raise blood sugar levels; for example, you could just eat meat. The trouble here is that your body needs glucose, but just not too much. Also, eating very high amounts of animal protein, especially from red meat, is bad for your kidneys and your bones and is associated with an increased colon-cancer risk. It's an extreme. Perhaps it's a useful direction to go in the short-term but not a good long-term diet. That's the Atkins-type diet direction. Another way is simply to eat carbohydrate foods that release their sugar content more slowly. These, as we have just seen, are called low-GI foods – for example, wholemeal brown bread instead of refined white. This is a step in the right direction, giving you a better 'quality' of carbohydrate foods, although you can still go overboard. In other words, you not only need to eat brown rather than white bread but less carbohydrate overall.

The GL score of a food already factors this in, so when you eat 45GLs a day you have automatically eaten both a lesser quantity of carbs and a better quality of them as far as your blood sugar is concerned. But you do also need to consciously eat a little more protein and healthy omega-3 fats.

4 Only eat carbs with protein You don't just need to eat more protein and healthy fat overall; you also need to eat it whenever you eat carbohydrate, because this helps to release the carbohydrate slowly. So, egg and sugar-free beans is in, whereas jam on toast is out. If you have an apple, you must have, for example, some nuts or seeds. The reason for this is that even if a food has a particular GL score, eating it with protein lowers the GL of the meal. The GL score for strawberries, for example, was initially worked out by feeding volunteers strawberries on their own and measuring what effect it had on their blood sugar level. But when you eat strawberries with yoghurt, for example, the protein takes longer to digest, so the sugars in the strawberries are also released more slowly, further lowering the GL of the meal.

Anything that slows down the release of sugars in foods lowers the GL. The combination of proteins with healthy fats will also help lower the GL score of your meal. In the next chapter I'm going to tell you about some amazing fibres that, if you add a teaspoonful to your meal, will automatically lower the GL.

Now that you know the 'rules' you could jump straight to Part 4 and get on with the diet if you like, but it's a good idea to understand why these rules exist and why eating my low-GL diet is the ultimate way to control your blood sugar.

In case you are wondering, this is not a difficult diet to do and soon becomes a habit. You don't get hungry, your energy increases and there are many side-benefits, including rapid weight loss if this is what you need.

CHAPTER 9

Why Stress Really Matters

If you ask the man or woman in the street whether stress is an important factor in heart disease just about everyone will agree. Even your doctor will say it's important to reduce your stress, but being hard to measure, unlike your cholesterol level, it's one of those factors that's given lip service but rather sidelined both in the treatment of heart disease and in research, precisely because there isn't a simple and accepted objective 'stress test', nor a profitable drug to treat it.

Yet stress has very precise ways of affecting your cardiovascular system, and there are also very precise ways to reduce your stress reaction. Understanding how stress could affect you helps to explain why other diet and lifestyle habits that switch on stress hormones, such as smoking cigarettes, and those that switch it off, such as exercise and drinking alcohol in moderation, can reduce your risk.

The effects of stress are often underestimated

First, let's look at some of the evidence that puts stress on the map. As part of the massive international INTERHEART study, which investigated risk factors for heart disease by comparing those who have it with those who don't, Professor Annika Rosengren said, in an interview in the *Telegraph*, that 'Severe stress makes it two and a half times more likely that an individual will have a heart attack. The

INTERHEART study shows that stress is one of the most important factors in heart attack in all ethnic groups and in all countries.'[41] Their study had found that psychosocial factors were responsible for about a third of the risk of heart disease.[42] But this might be an underestimate, because other important risk factors such as smoking, a lack of exercise and moderate drinking of alcohol (which reduces risk) might also be partly working because of a stress reduction effect.

The other factors they found that increased risk were being diabetic, having abdominal weight gain, having high blood pressure and a high apoB/ApoA-1 ratio (which is equivalent to a high LDL/HDL ratio).

In the last chapter we learnt that as you lose blood sugar control you get sugar highs and lows. These lows trigger the release of stress hormones, notably cortisol, which makes you more stressed, whereas the removed blood sugar, now stored in the liver where it is turned into fat, then gets dumped around your middle. A consequence, seen in diabetics, is increased LDL and reduced HDL. These measures, together with high blood pressure, are not original 'causes' of heart disease but rather consequences of something you do or don't do, be it, for example, eating a high-GL diet or a diet deficient in magnesium. I discuss magnesium deficiency in depth in Chapter 13; but even magnesium deficiency itself could be a consequence of stress, because a high stress level is known to cause magnesium excretion.

Dr Malcolm Kendrick, author of *The Great Cholesterol Con*, argues that many of the patterns of change in the incidence of heart disease could also be explained by stress. This includes 'low risk' nationalities moving into Western countries – when they do so, up goes their risk. This is often attributed to adopting a Western lifestyle and diet, such as the Japanese living in America, but perhaps emigrating, and what happened to cause the emigration, plays a big part too. Kendrick gives many examples of dislocation leading to massive increases in heart disease rate and in big social upheavals. One example is the massive unemployment in Glasgow from the 1940s to the 1960s, leading to relocation to some dismal places

– potential factors for Glasgow becaming the UK's capital of heart attacks. Of course, it is hard to definitively 'prove' what does what. Also bear in mind that the lack of a blood test to diagnose 'stress' and the slim prospect of a profitable drug to treat it means that the effects of stress are not given the attention they deserve.

Why how you feel matters

Furthermore, although measuring cholesterol is 'objective', measures of stress levels, such as in the INTERHEART research, are done by asking people questions, and this is therefore 'subjective', which many scientists don't like. As a psychologist I have no problem with collecting 'subjective' information. After all, you are more likely to know how you feel than anyone else.

Other studies using 'subjective' measures of stress have reported that too much stress can be as bad for your heart as smoking and high cholesterol[43] and increase your risk of dying from heart-related problems five-fold.[44] In our 100% Health Survey,[45] 68 per cent of the 55,000-plus participants reported feeling that they have too much to do, 66 per cent said they frequently felt anxious or tense, 82 per cent often became impatient and 55 per cent got angry easily.

Defining stress

Stress is a term we use when we are under too much pressure. As life gets faster and faster, and it's harder to make a living, many of us live in a semi-permanent state of stress. Significant changes, health problems, relationship and money problems are common causes of stress; however, it's the daily pressure we feel in response to everyday hassles – like being stuck in traffic, experiencing delays in getting things sorted and receiving too many emails – that does as much damage.

Stress is both the body's and the mind's response to any pressure that disrupts our equilibrium. It occurs when your perception of events doesn't meet your expectations and you are unable to manage your reaction. Our response to stressful events is one of resistance, tension, anxiety and frustration that throws off our physiological and psychological balance, with increased pulse, higher levels of adrenal hormones, inhibition of digestion and all sorts of other changes that, from an evolutionary point of view, gear you up for 'fight or flight'. Prolonged stress has severe consequences, locking your physiology into an unhealthy state that increases your risk of heart disease. Many of us think we get used to this stress state, living with a low-grade state of anxiety, but, insidiously, stress does its damage.

Stress changes what you eat

One of the ways we deal with stress is to eat comfort food, drink alcohol or use caffeine or sugar to keep going. These are coping mechanisms that, in turn, increase your cardiovascular risk. In a poll, 46 per cent of people, when stressed, said they were less careful about their food choices. Some don't eat, others eat lots of carbs and sugar or fatty foods. Researchers at Ohio State University found that short periods of emotional stress can slow down the body's process of clearing some fats from the bloodstream, possibly contributing to heart disease.

Stress also depletes the body of many nutrients, particularly magnesium, which helps to relax both your mind and your arteries. So, when stressed, it is especially important to eat well, yet we often compound the problem by doing exactly the opposite.

How stress affects your heart

According to the American Institute of Stress, up to 90 per cent of all health problems are related to stress. Too much stress can contribute to many health problems including heart disease, high blood pressure, stroke, depression and sleeping problems.

Learning from the research

Many studies confirm the debilitating effects of stress on our health:

- Three 10-year studies concluded that emotional stress was more predictive of death from cancer and cardiovascular disease than smoking. People who were unable to effectively manage their stress had a 40 per cent higher death rate than non-stressed individuals.[46]
- A Harvard Medical School study of 1,623 heart attack survivors found that when subjects got angry during emotional conflicts, their risk of subsequent heart attacks was more than double that of those who remained calm.[47]
- A 20-year study of over 1,700 older men conducted by the Harvard School of Public Health found that worry about social conditions, health and personal finances all significantly increased the risk of coronary heart disease.[48]
- According to a Mayo Clinic study of individuals with heart disease, psychological stress was the strongest predictor of future cardiac events, such as cardiac death, cardiac arrest and heart attacks.[49]

The science behind exactly how high levels of stress affect the heart and arteries has come a long way and now there actually are objective ways of measuring it.

Stress has the opposite effect of relaxation. When you are relaxed, this turns on a pattern of nervous-system activity, called the parasympathetic nervous system, which slows your heart rate, reduces your blood pressure and does good things to your arteries (see the illustration 'How your emotional state reflects chemical and hormonal stress levels' on page 100).

When you are stressed, this does the opposite by switching on what's called the sympathetic nervous system (which is the opposite of sympathetic to your heart). Up go your blood pressure and your blood sugar and your heart beats rapidly. On a chemical level you produce more adrenalin and cortisol and, with this, your HDL goes down and LDL goes up, then out pour all sorts of clotting factors. Why?

Stress is part of the 'fight/flight' syndrome. Your system is getting ready to fight, forcing more oxygen and glucose around the system with more blood pressure for the anticipated burst of activity, and preparing your system for injury by clotting the blood in case you get cut. All good stuff if you are charging into battle, but inappropriate if you are sitting there on a Monday morning thinking about going to do a job you don't want to do, while having a cigarette and a coffee to give you some get up and go. No wonder heart attacks are much more common on a Monday morning.

The counter-hormone to cortisol is DHEA, also produced by the adrenal glands. By measuring not just the level of cortisol and DHEA but their pattern over 20 hours, it is possible to get a good sense as to how stressed a person is. But there's another way, based on the effect of sympathetic versus parasympathetic nervous activity.

Heart-rate variability: an excellent indicator of stress

At a very basic level you could say that stress raises your heartbeat, so higher heartbeat presumably means more stress – but so too does running for the bus. More significant is the pattern of what happens between heartbeats. This is called your heart-rate variability, or HRV, which is now an accepted measure of your state of stress or negative emotion. You can measure this with a simple handheld device against which you put your thumb to pick up the heartbeat signal.

When you are not stressed, and are in a more open, positive state of mind, you get a different pattern of HRV, called high 'coherence'. On a graph it looks like hills (see first graph on page 99). In a state of stress your HRV graph is much more erratic (see second graph on page 99). (In Chapter 24 I'm going to show you some simple 'HeartMath' techniques that can help you quickly switch out of a stress reaction in difficult moments.)

Although this is in its infancy, studies measuring HRV, and also employing these HeartMath techniques to reduce stress, are proving very promising indeed in reducing heart disease risk.

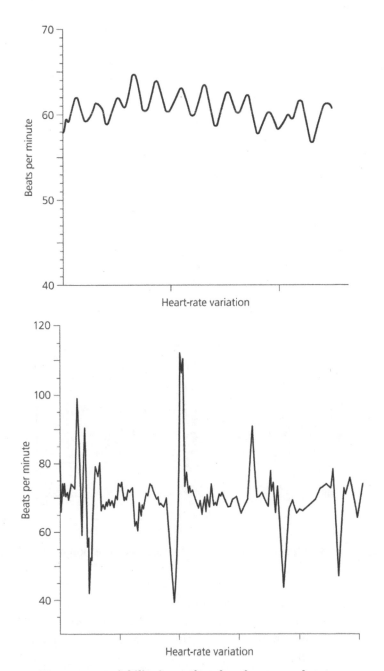

Heart-rate variability in a relaxed and a stressed state

The opposite of stress is not necessarily being super-relaxed. You can be firing on all cylinders and in a positive emotional state, but although your sympathetic nervous system activity is high, you don't have high cortisol. This is a state of 'positive stress', where you are coping well and enjoying a challenging situation. High achievers who enjoy their jobs often spend a lot of time in this top right quadrant in the illustration below.

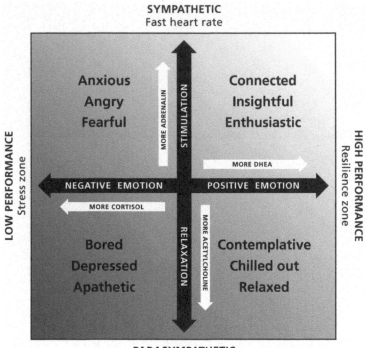

How your emotional state reflects chemical and hormonal stress levels

What you want to avoid is being in the top left quadrant: stressed and unhappy, with emotions such as anger, irritation, frustration, fear and anxiety. These are the negative emotional states that increase your risk of a heart attack.

How balancing your HRV reduces your risk

Numerous studies have shown that regularly practising HeartMath can be hugely beneficial for your heart. In one study, after just one month, cortisol (the stress hormone) was reduced by 23 per cent and DHEA (the healthy hormone) increased by 100 per cent.[50]

In a study on patients with high blood pressure, their blood pressure dropped substantially after three months by using the HeartMath techniques, along with improvements in emotional health.[51] On average their blood pressure dropped by 10.6/6.3 points. In a group of 75 patients with abnormal heart rhythms (atrial fibrillation) the study noted that they were substantially improved after three months and 14 were able to discontinue medication altogether.[52] Other studies have shown these techniques to be very effective in reducing stress levels in those with heart disease.[53]

Other stress-reduction techniques reported highly positive effects. An eight-year study, published in *Archives of Internal Medicine*,[54] looked at the effects of meditation on stress and heart disease and found it cut the risk of a heart attack, stroke or death and also lowered systolic blood pressure by around 4.9mmHg more than in the control group. Just ten or twenty minutes of meditation, once or twice a day, was highly effective in more than halving risk. Dr Schneider, who conducted the study, said:

> These findings are the strongest documented effects yet produced by a mind-body intervention on cardiovascular disease. They indicate that stress reduction with the transcendental meditation technique is an effective approach in the prevention of heart disease. This study builds on previous research findings showing that the Transcendental Meditation program reduces high blood pressure, high cholesterol, insulin resistance, psychological stress, and atherosclerosis, and takes it to the next step – lower rates of death, heart attack, and stroke.'

Summary

Reducing your stress level is a very important and highly effective way of reducing your risk of heart disease, lowering your blood pressure and improving recovery from heart disease. Often we look at outside events as the source of stress, but in fact stress is really caused by our own emotional reactions to events.

While there are practical steps you can take to reduce your stress levels, one of the most important skills to learn is how to master your own stress response the moment it occurs, or in preparation for a potentially stressful situation. In Part 4 I'll be showing you how to assess your stress level, the factors that cause your stress and how you can start to reduce and master your own stress response. This is a vital piece of the healthy heart equation.

CHAPTER 10

How High is Your Homocysteine?

One of the most fundamental biochemical balancing acts going on in your body is something called methylation. It's how the body makes and balances thousands of biochemicals. There are approximately a billion of these methylation reactions every few seconds, making sure you stay in good health.

The raw material for doing all this methylation is a dietary amino acid called methionine. It is converted into the methylation hero, s-adenosyl methionine (SAMe), by enzymes that depend on B vitamins, especially B_6, B_{12} and folic acid, plus a few other nutrients. If you don't have enough of these nutrients, your homocysteine level starts to rise and the higher it goes the greater your risk of heart disease becomes.

If you're at risk of cardiovascular disease, or have a family history of heart disease or stroke, it is essential that your doctor checks your homocysteine level. There's no question that having a raised homocysteine level is a significant and independent risk factor for cardiovascular disease – both heart attacks and strokes.

In relation to strokes, a study, published in 2001, showed that a raised homocysteine level is a better predictor of cardiovascular problems than a stroke victim's age (each additional year adds only a 6 per cent risk), blood pressure, cholesterol level or whether or not they smoked.[55] The study involved 1,158 women and 789 men aged 60 years or older who had already taken part in studies investigating homocysteine levels as a predictor for stroke. After seven years, those who had had a homocysteine score above 14mcmol/l had an 82 per cent increased risk of stroke, compared to those with less than 9.2. If your level is slightly raised (5 points higher than normal) you'll increase your risk of a heart attack by 42 per cent, of deep vein thrombosis by 60 per cent and of a stroke by 65 per cent, according to a meta-analysis of 92 studies in the *British Medical Journal*.[56] 'These results provide strong evidence that the association between homocysteine and cardiovascular disease is causal,' says lead author, David Wald, Clinical Research Fellow in Cardiology at the Wolfson Institute of Preventive Medicine at Barts in London.

The value of checking your homocysteine

More recent studies continue to confirm that homocysteine is an independent predictor of risk. Among elderly people, for example, cholesterol is a very poor predictor of cardiovascular disease death, as is the widely used index of conventional risk factors called the Framingham Risk Score that I mentioned in Part I; the Framingham Risk Score involves an equation based on your blood pressure, cholesterol, ECG, diabetes risk and whether you smoke. According to a study published in the *British Medical Journal*, the best predictor by far is your homocysteine: a level above 13mcmol/l predicted no fewer than two-thirds of all deaths five years on.[57] Another finds that having a homocysteine level above 15mcmol/l more than doubles your risk of cardiovascular disease or having, or dying from, a cardiovascular event.[58]

To put this into context, the average adult in Britain has a homocysteine level of around 11 mcmol/l, compared to an ideal level below 7. Most people are already at risk, according to their homocysteine levels.

Why does raised homocysteine increase risk?

The homocysteine theory was first proposed in 1969 by Dr Kilmer McCully, a pathologist at the VA Medical Center in Providence,

Rhode Island, USA. He had been studying a rare genetic disorder called homocysteinuria. Children born with this condition lack certain enzymes required to turn the toxic substance homocysteine into harmless cystanthionine. Unless they are diagnosed and treated, these children often die of heart attacks and strokes before reaching adulthood, induced by thrombosis, despite having completely normal cholesterol levels.

Although the genetic disease homocysteinuria is rare, McCully wondered what percentage of people produced small excesses of homocysteine which, over many years, might increase their risk. He also wondered to what extent homocysteine excess was limited to those with a genetic predisposition or whether it could occur in anyone lacking vitamins B_6, B_{12} or folic acid, deficiencies of which are extremely common.

As his investigation unfolded he found that smoking and inactivity tended to raise homocysteine levels and that those people with a family history of heart disease often shared a minor flaw in one of the genes governing homocysteine metabolism.

Homocysteine levels rise with age; women have, on average, 20 per cent lower levels than men, until the menopause after which levels between the sexes are more or less equal. All of these findings fitted perfectly with the incidence of heart attacks occurring more often in smoking, sedentary men, and then rising in women after the menopause. It was also well known that injecting animals with homocysteine produces arterial plaque.

How does homocysteine cause heart disease?

Excess homocysteine in your blood is toxic to arteries and could cause the initial damage to the artery wall that starts the whole process of cardiovascular disease. Also, excess homocysteine, partly by being converted into a substance called homocysteine thiolactone, encourages thrombosis.[59] This is thought to combine with LDL, producing an abnormal molecule that the immune system's macrophages attack, producing foam cells, fatty streaks and atherosclerosis, in much the same way that oxidised LDL cholesterol does (see page 28). When homocysteine goes up, HDL cholesterol goes down. It promotes inflammation and also lowers the level of NO (nitric oxide), which improves blood flow and relaxes arteries.[60] Many drugs given for heart disease and high blood pressure work by raising NO (more on this on page 186.)[61] This combination of factors is likely to explain why high homocysteine would increase arterial disease.[62] Also, since a high homocysteine level means poor methylation, and since methylation actually controls genetic expression, another possibility is that homocysteine pushes genetic expression towards disease.[63] When combined with increased oxidation, this makes a person with a high homocysteine score a prime candidate for a stroke or heart attack.[64]

Proving the homocysteine theory

It wasn't until the 1990s that the evidence for the homocysteine theory started to become very convincing.[65] In 1992 a study of 14,000 male doctors found that those in the top 5 per cent of homocysteine levels had three times the heart attack risk, compared to those in the bottom 5 per cent. This increased risk was confirmed by the Massachusetts-based Framingham Heart Study in 1995, which found that having more than 11.4mcmol/l of homocysteine in the blood increased the risk.[66] Another study, at the University of Washington, found that having high homocysteine doubles the risk of heart attack in young women.

The real clincher was a study carried out by the European Concerted Action Group, a consortium of doctors and researchers from 19 medical centres in nine European countries.[67] They studied 750 people under the age of 60 with atherosclerosis, compared to 800 people without such cardiovascular disease. They found that having a high level of homocysteine in the blood was as great a risk factor for cardiovascular disease as smoking or having a high blood cholesterol level. Those in the top fifth of homocysteine levels had double the risk of cardiovascular disease. In other words, 20 per cent of people had double the risk of cardiovascular disease because of high homocysteine levels. A meta-analysis of all studies up to 2008 concludes, 'each increase of 5µmol/L in homocysteine levels increases the risk of CHD events by approximately 20 per cent, independently of traditional CHD risk factors'.[68]

The European Concerted Action Group also found that those taking vitamin supplements reduced their risk to a third of those not taking supplements. When they compared blood levels of vitamins B_6, B_{12} and folic acid, they found that there was a direct relationship between increasing homocysteine levels with decreasing levels of folic acid and vitamin B_6, with vitamin B_6 having the strongest association. In this study B_{12} status didn't correlate with homocysteine levels.

By the late 1990s leading cardiovascular researchers were recommending higher levels of these vitamins than can easily be gained from diet alone, namely at least 10–50mg of vitamin B_6 and 400–1,000mcg of folic acid, plus 10mcg of B_{12}. As *Newsweek* reported in August 1997, 'It may turn out that we can achieve more with nickel-and-dime vitamin supplements than with drugs that cost hundreds of times more.'

Mixed evidence

If you suggest this to your doctor, however, he or she may reply that several large trials have found that lowering homocysteine doesn't reduce your risk of heart attacks or a stroke. In the last decade a number of studies, but not all, that have given high-dose B vitamins, usually to those who have a high risk or who have had a cardiovascular event such as a heart attack, have seen reductions in homocysteine but not a reduced risk of, for example, a second heart attack. A review of eight studies concludes, 'homocysteine-lowering interventions do not reduce the risk of non-fatal or fatal myocardial infarction, stroke, or death by any cause'.[69]

Although it is true that giving homocysteine-lowering B vitamins to people who have heart disease has been disappointing, it appears that giving them to those without heart disease does reduce risk. Fortification of flour with folic acid (an important homocysteine-lowering B vitamin) in Canada and the US has coincided with a considerable drop in heart attack and stroke rates of between 10 and 15 per cent. Translated into UK terms, that means that increasing folic acid intake could actually save more than 5,000 lives a year.

Particularly where strokes are concerned, lowering homocysteine by taking folic acid makes a big difference. It can lower stroke risk by 31 per cent, according to another analysis of trials published in the *Lancet*.[70]

On the other hand, a study in the *American Journal of Cardiology* found that cardiovascular patients with high homocysteine levels (above 15mcmol/l) who were treated with B vitamins cut their risk of death by a quarter over ten years. Among those not given the B vitamins 32 per cent had died, compared to only 4 per cent of those given high-dose vitamins. This means that those on placebo were eight times more likely to die than those on B vitamins. So why the different results?

Why have B vitamins failed to reduce risk in some studies?

There are a few possibilities. A lay person would probably assume that the people studied in the eight ineffective studies, 24,210 in all, had high homocysteine levels to start with and that they were given a combination of the known B vitamins that most effectively lower homocysteine. This, however, was not the case.

A high homocysteine level is usually defined as above 15mcmol/l; however, none of these study populations had averages above this. Two of the eight studies didn't even report homocysteine levels. Those that did ranged between scores of 11.2 and 13.4, which is certainly not ideal, but not very high. The average person in Britain is probably between 9 and 12. That's a bit like giving statins to people without high cholesterol levels. It's not surprising not much happened. (The same is true with statins.)

Some people, however, have homocysteine levels from 15 to over a 100. These are the people who are likely to benefit most from homocysteine-lowering B vitamins. That's what the research shows.

The next critical question is: were the vitamins given effective in lowering only moderately raised homocysteine levels? Three studies didn't even report follow-up tests, so we are left with five studies. Averaged, they produced a 20 per cent drop in homocysteine. So, the average starting point is 12.4mcmol/l, which is not very high, and the ending point is 10mcmol/l, which is not very different. To put this in context, when I have patients with homocysteine levels above 15mcmol/l, I expect to bring them down by at least 50 per cent within three months.

We have to ask why were the interventions in these studies rather ineffective in lowering homocysteine and lowering risk? The nutrients that do effectively lower homocysteine are vitamins B_6, folic acid, B_{12}, and also zinc with tri-methyl-glycine (TMG) in the right doses. The least effective drop was achieved in the CHAOS study, which gave only folic acid. The two most effective (Norvit and Wafacs) gave the most vitamin B_{12} (1,000mcg). None gave zinc and TMG. Also, folic acid fortification was just starting in the US and it is possible that the people studied (in both the vitamin and the placebo groups) might not have been particularly lacking in these vitamins.

Taking drugs affects B vitamins' effectiveness

Of course, another factor is that most of the people in these trials were also on a plethora of cardiovascular drugs, and it is possible that this interfered with the ability of the B vitamins to do anything positive.

Homocysteine prevents platelets sticking, which stops blood clots – something aspirin also does, so if people in the trials were already taking aspirin there would be no extra benefit in lowering homocysteine with B vitamins. Aspirin was in fact widely used by participants in the trials, because they were mainly conducted in patients who had already had a heart attack or other cardiovascular diseases.

Research led by Dr David Wald at the Wolfson Institute of Preventive Medicine at Barts and the London School of Medicine and Dentistry showed that there was a difference in the reduction in heart disease events between the five trials with the lowest aspirin use (60 per cent of the participants took aspirin) and the five trials with the highest use (91 per cent took aspirin).[71] The observed risk reduction was 6 per cent, but it would have been 15 per cent if no one had been taking aspirin. Research was based on 75 epidemiological studies involving about 50,000 participants and clinical trials involving about 40,000 participants.

'The explanation has important implications,' said Dr Wald, the lead author of the paper. 'The negative clinical trial evidence should not close the door on folic acid – folic acid may still be of benefit in people who have not had a heart attack because they will generally not be taking aspirin.' Unlike aspirin, which damages the gut, the potential side effects of B vitamins are better memory and mood. Of course, aspirin isn't the only drug given in these trials. Most people were on five different medications that could have rendered the B vitamins they took ineffective. One recent critique of the failed studies says, 'The protocols neglected an essential fact: that the impact of some confounding factors, such as concomitant use of statins, acetylsalicylic acid, folic acid, and other drugs, might have led to bias and an inappropriate interpretation of the data. The cardiovascular protective and preventive effects of statins and aspirin might have reduced or abolished the possibility of observing a difference in the number of events between the vitamin and placebo groups for the clinical endpoints.' A further study, re-analysing the apparent lack of effect of B vitamins, reached the same conclusion – that antiplatelet drugs such as aspirin stop B vitamins working.[72,73] Don't give up on B vitamins for heart protection, they conclude. Better-designed studies are clearly needed.

Test your homocysteine

The important point is to test your homocysteine level, rather than just take high-dose B vitamins. If it is above 15mcmol/l you are highly likely to benefit from lowering your homocysteine. If it is above 10 you really need to lower it (a level above 10mcmol/l equates to accelerated brain shrinkage, and probably bone shrinkage). Below this it is not clear what benefit you'll get, but I would recommend getting it to below 7 for optimal health. If your doctor won't test you, you can do it yourself with a home-test kit (see Resources). Here's how to lower it:

- Eat more vegetable protein from seeds, nuts and beans (these are rich in folic acid)

- Eat more greens (also rich in folic acid)

- Cut back on coffee (two coffees raise homocysteine by 14 per cent in four hours)

- Limit alcohol

- Reduce stress

- Stop smoking

- Supplement homocysteine-lowering nutrients daily

The most effective way is to supplement a homocysteine-lowering formula that contains not only B_6, B_{12} and folic acid but also B_2, zinc, TMG and n-acetyl cysteine (NAC). This combination is the most effective for lowering homocysteine fast. How much you need depends on your homocysteine level, and this is explained in Part 4 (see page 237).

Summary

- Take high-dose vitamin C, lysine and niacin as described in Chapter 22.
- Test your homocysteine level. If it is above 15mcmol/l you are highly likely to benefit from lowering your homocysteine.
- Lower high homocysteine by eating vegetable protein from seeds, nuts and beans, green leafy vegetables, reducing coffee, limiting alcohol, stopping smoking and finding ways to reduce stress.
- See Part 4, page 237 for details of how to supplement a homocysteine-lowering formula that contains vitamins B_6, B_{12} and folic acid, B_2, zinc, TMG and NAC.

Chapter 22 helps you build your own supplement programme.

CHAPTER 11

Lipoprotein(a), Niacin and Vitamin C

T he chances are you've never heard of lipoprotein(a) and never been tested for it. Lipoprotein(a) is a particularly sticky fat, a relative of LDL, that binds to artery walls producing a thickening of arterial plaque. Like LDL cholesterol, it is an independent and reliable marker of heart disease and is considered to be part of the cause, not just an indicator of risk. The higher your level the greater your risk.[73]

Lipoprotein(a) is heading for inclusion as an important risk factor for heart disease, along with homocysteine, and one that should be checked. It can be lowered, not with drugs but with B vitamins.

A recent study in the journal *Thrombosis Research*[74] involving 955 people who had coronary artery disease, many of whom had suffered a heart attack, found that knowing a woman's lipoprotein(a) (which is abbreviated to Lp(a)) and homocysteine predicted risk to a significant level, although this is not the case in men. Having both an elevated homocysteine and Lp(a) 'conferred a significant, 3.6-fold risk of coronary artery disease in females and an even higher 11-fold risk in young females, which suggested an interactive effect' say the authors. It is becoming considered an independent and causal risk factor in heart disease.

A meta-study of 27 studies following up people over an average period of 10 years found that those in the top third of Lp(a) levels, with levels above 100mg/dl, were at a 70 per cent increased risk of coronary heart disease risk compared with subjects in the lowest third, with an average level of 5mg/dL.[75] Top European cardiovascular experts recommend that anyone with an Lp(a) level above 50mg/dl should be treated, not with drugs but with vitamins;[76] however, it would appear that optimum levels are below 10mg/dl. This is not a routine test but certainly one any good cardiologist would be familiar with.

What your lipoprotein(a) level indicates

Low risk	Medium	High	Very High
10mg/dl	20mg/dl	30mg/dl	50mg/dl

The vitamin C–lipoprotein(a) story

Back in the 1950s a Canadian doctor, C.G. Willis, discovered that guinea pigs deprived of sufficient vitamin C produced atherosclerotic plaque. Then, in the 1990s, Dr Linus Pauling (a scientific genius with two Nobel Prizes to his name) and his colleagues proposed that the development of cardiovascular disease, the number-one killer in the Western world, may have prevented our extinction. Their paper 'A Unified Theory of Human Cardiovascular Disease' attracted considerable interest among leading cardiologists.[77]

Their theory was that the formation of lipoprotein(a) was a consequence of a lack of vitamin C. In case you didn't know this, all animals, with the exception of guinea pigs, fruit-eating bats, the red-vented bulbul bird and primates, make vitamin C in their bodies. The amount varies from creature to creature but it is usually in the human equivalent of a range of 1,000–20,000mg per day. Most people in the Western world currently consume below 100mg. About 40 million years ago the ancestor of humankind lost this ability to synthesise vitamin C from glucose and, as a result, we now depend entirely on dietary sources. The probable reason why such a genetic mutation occurred was that we had sufficient supplies in our diet. Indeed, our ancestors' diet, being rich in fruits and other plant material, could easily have provided several grams per day. When our ancestors left tropical regions, however, to settle in other parts of the world (especially during the Ice Age, when vegetation was very scarce) they would have been at a high risk of developing scurvy, caused by vitamin C deficiency.

Scurvy is a fatal disease. It is characterised by a breakdown of the connective tissue in the body. Ascorbate (vitamin C) is essential in the production of collagen and elastin, which bind together the skin, membranes and cells. The first sign of scurvy is vascular bleeding: as blood vessels start to leak, their membranes are under more pressure than any other part of the body, because of the force of blood pumping through them. In the 19th century, blood loss from scurvy decimated ship crews. It is quite conceivable that death from scurvy could have decimated the human species, especially during the thousands of years of the Ice Ages.

Nature on the defensive

So how did we survive? According to Pauling we may have developed the ability to deposit lipids (fats) along the artery walls to protect them from deteriorating and bleeding in order to increase our chances of surviving during ascorbate-deficient times.[78]

Another group of proteins (which normally accumulate at injury sites to effect repair) are fibrinogen and apoprotein. Lipids and apoprotein combine to produce lipoprotein(a) which, in excess, is a good predictor of impending cardiovascular disease.

Lipoprotein(a) can repair damaged or leaky blood vessels, but it also increases the risk of heart disease by building up deposits on artery walls.[79] Pauling proposed that a lack of vitamin C would lead to an increase in lipoprotein(a), which would, in effect, stop the arteries leaking. Could this have been nature's answer to life-threatening scurvy? If so, does taking large amounts of vitamin C reverse heart disease?

Taking high-dose vitamin C makes a lot of sense because it does lower LDL cholesterol when given to healthy people,[80] diabetics[81] and people on kidney dialysis,[82] and it has also been shown to reduce arterial thickening.[83] It is also an anti-inflammatory and may help,

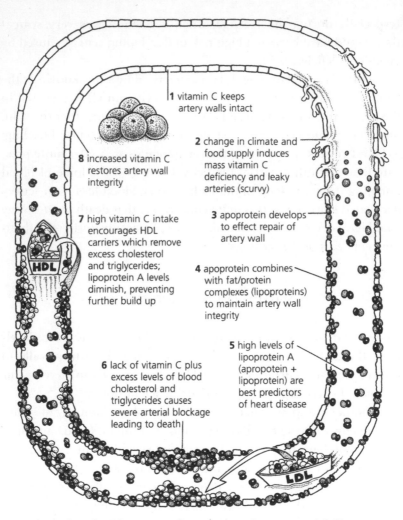

1 vitamin C keeps artery walls intact

2 change in climate and food supply induces mass vitamin C deficiency and leaky arteries (scurvy)

8 increased vitamin C restores artery wall integrity

3 apoprotein develops to effect repair of artery wall

7 high vitamin C intake encourages HDL carriers which remove excess cholesterol and triglycerides; lipoprotein A levels diminish, preventing further build up

4 apoprotein combines with fat/protein complexes (lipoproteins) to maintain artery wall integrity

HDL

5 high levels of lipoprotein A (apropotein + lipoprotein) are best predictors of heart disease

6 lack of vitamin C plus excess levels of blood cholesterol and triglycerides causes severe arterial blockage leading to death

LDL

How vitamin C is proposed to cause and cure arterial disease

together with vitamin E, to stop the oxidation, or damage, of cholesterol.[84] A recent study of almost 60,000 people in Japan reports that vitamin C intake is strongly associated with a reduced risk of heart disease, especially in women, cutting risk by a third.[85] Another reports that vitamin C, with vitamin E, slows down atherosclerosis.[86] It also lowers blood pressure.[87] Many diet studies also find that the higher your dietary intake of vitamin C the lower your risk.

Although high-dose vitamin C does appear to reduce cardio-vascular risk, however, it does not appear to consistently lower lipoprotein(a). One research group gave 4.5g a day for 12 weeks and found no significant change.[88] Vitamin C on its own doesn't seem to be the magic bullet but, together with other nutrients, it is well worth considering if you have heart disease.

Lysine stops lipoproteins binding to your arteries

Pauling and colleagues proposed that the solution to stopping lipoprotein(a) binding to the arteries was to give both high-dose vitamin C together with the amino acid lysine, which inhibits lipoprotein(a) sticking to artery walls. They recommended something in the region of 5–10g of vitamin C with 3–6g of lysine and published some very impressive case histories of atherosclerotic plaque reversal and relief from angina.[89] One such case is of a leading US biochemist who had had three coronary bypass operations, numerous complications and angina (heart pain) at the slightest exertion. He took many daily medications including beta blockers and aspirin. His cardiologist confirmed that a fourth coronary bypass operation was not possible, and he advised him to add to his medication 6g of ascorbic acid, 60mg of CoQ_{10}, a multivitamin tablet with minerals, additional vitamins A, E and B complex, lecithin and niacin (B_3). Linus Pauling recommended he continue the ascorbic acid and add 5g of lysine daily.

The biochemist started with 1g of lysine in May 1991, and increased the daily dose to 5g by mid-June. By mid-July he could walk two miles and do gardening work without angina pain and wrote, 'The effects of the lysine borders on the miraculous.' He attributed his newfound well-being to the addition of lysine and vitamins to his other medications.

A patient of mine, who had had three strokes and had suffered from high blood pressure for ten years, came to me suffering from angina due to a blocked coronary artery. Even a brisk walk gave him extreme chest pain. He took 5g of vitamin C and 3g of lysine, plus 600ius of vitamin E and 30mg of CoQ_{10}. Five months later, having stopped taking two drugs for high blood pressure, his blood pressure was normal and he could raise his exercising pulse rate up to 180 beats per minute before experiencing any pain.

Another patient who had suffered a major heart attack was left unable to walk up any incline due to severe angina. Within three months on vitamin C and lysine he was able to walk up hills again.

Another man who believes Linus Pauling helped him to recover from disablement and the brink of death is David Holmes. Writing in the journal *Holistic Health*,[90] he told his story. 'At the age of 48 I had a sudden and quite severe heart attack with no prior warning symptoms.' After that he devised an excellent nutritional prevention strategy.

All went very well for about seventeen years. But in August 1993 I began to suffer from angina pains when making very short walks of some 20 yards. My blood tests showed that my blood chemistry was normal in most respects: low in cholesterol, high in HDL. My blood analysis also showed something else. It showed a dangerously high lipoprotein(a). I began taking 1g L-lysine and 1g vitamin C in three separate doses thrice daily. Over three weeks I increased these amounts up to a total of 6g lysine and 6g vitamin C. Other supplements I added were omega-3 fatty acids and magnesium. On this new regime my angina became less and less frequent and my exercise tolerance increased as the days went by. Subsequent blood tests showed a dramatic fall in both lipoprotein(a) and apolipoprotein A2 (another potentially harmful lipoprotein). Having reduced both the lipoprotein (a) and apolipoprotein A2 to normal, the angina became much less frequent so that some three months after beginning I was able to go to the Maritime Alps and walk three to six miles per day up and down the mountains without pain for three weeks at Christmas time. Finally, I was able to stop the beta-blocker Atenolol and Diltiazem completely.

Extraordinarily, in the past 20 years no clinical trial has been done on the combination of lysine and vitamin C so this theory remains unproven. Linus Pauling died in his nineties shortly after publishing his paper, so further research on these inexpensive and non-patentable nutrients depends on other research groups getting interested.

There is certainly good logic, however, to giving lysine to stop the binding of lipoproteins and presumably cholesterol to the arteries. There is growing evidence that this actually works in animal studies, but it hasn't been put to the test in human trials. Combining it with other heart-friendly nutrients may work even better.

Lipoprotein binding increases with increasing inflammation, which any of the diet and supplementary recommendations in this book, including increasing your intake of vitamin C, serve to reduce.[91,92]

Niacin lowers lipoprotein(a) as well as cholesterol

Although we are going to have to wait and see whether the combined effect of high-dose vitamin C and lysine develops, another vitamin is already proven to lower both cholesterol and lipoprotein(a) more effectively than any drug. It is niacin, vitamin B_3. As well as lowering cholesterol and raising HDL cholesterol, niacin is more effective than any drug for lowering lipoprotein(a), lowering high levels by about a third when high doses of niacin, 1g or more, are given for several months. One study from the King Gustav V Research Institute in Sweden reported a 37 per cent decrease in six weeks with high-dose niacin, given at a dose of 4 grams a day.[93] Other studies have shown the same thing, and a recent review concludes that no drugs really do this effectively and that 'the strongest effects are seen with niacin at high doses.'[94]

Vitamin B_3 (niacin) is usually given in doses of 1,000–2,000mg, in a non-blushing or slow-release form because, in high doses, it causes vasodilation (dilation of the blood vessels).

There are many good reasons to supplement high-dose niacin, which is available on prescription and in health-food stores. According to a major review of what works, in the *New England*

Journal of Medicine, 'the most effective way' to lower cholesterol is with niacin, not statin drugs.[95]

A number of studies show that it is effective not only in raising the good HDL by as much as 35 per cent but also in reducing LDL by up to 25 per cent. By way of comparison, statins only raise HDL by between 2 per cent and 15 per cent. Niacin also reduces levels of two other markers for heart disease – lipoprotein(a) and fibrinogen – the latter of which is also involved in binding lipoproteins to arteries.

The most obvious side effect of taking fairly high doses is a blushing effect, which is diminished by taking the nutrient with food; however, non-blush, or extended-release, niacin is now easily available. Other reported side effects include dyspepsia (indigestion), raised plasma glucose and uric acid levels, although these last two have not been confirmed in recent studies. Overall, it has nothing like the side effects associated with statins. Niacin was actually discovered to lower cholesterol back in the 1960s, as a 'side effect' of giving high doses to those with schizophrenia as a highly effective therapy pioneered by the late Dr Abram Hoffer. So it has taken 50 years for this discovery to come to market, largely because drug companies have explored ways of combining it with substances or processes that effectively 'slow release' it, which can be patented. You can buy straight niacin for very little, and although taking 500mg twice a day will produce major flushing for the first couple of days, the blushing soon diminishes as long as you keep going.

A recent big review of niacin trials found that because it had a 'markedly beneficial' effect on a particularly dangerous combination of risk factors – a low level of the good cholesterol HDL and high levels of triglyceride fats in the blood – it might be particularly useful in treating people who are heading towards diabetes.[96] Studies have shown that it inhibits atherosclerosis, reduces the risk of heart attack and, if taken over 15 years, lowers the risk of death.[97] The strongest evidence, however, has come from trials combining statins with niacin.[98] I suspect that, as the patents for statin drugs run out, the option of getting a patent for a combination of niacin plus a drug will be seen as one way to extend the process of making money from statins. All was going well until a study combining niacin with statins was stopped in 2011 because the niacin wasn't adding benefit to the drug regime.[99] Much like homocysteine, we may find that drugs dampen down or interfere with the ability of nutrients to make a difference. What we really need is a niacin vs. statin trial, but that's not in the interests of the pharmaceutical industry which makes lots of money from statins and which funds most of these trials.

If I had heart disease, I'd start by taking niacin instead of a statin. After all, it lowers LDL cholesterol, triglycerides and Lp(a), raises HDL, has clinical evidence of reducing risk of cardiovascular disease and death, and is a naturally occurring nutrient, with no side effects beyond the blushing effect. However, if you've had a heart attack, and statins have successfully lowered your cholesterol, and if you don't have too low an HDL level and you're not getting adverse reactions from the statins, then there's good reason to continue.

Summary

- To reduce your risk of cardiovascular problems, check your lipoprotein(a) level, which you will need to request, and probably pay for, via your cardiologist or health-care practitioner.
- If it is raised (above 30mg/dL) and especially if you also have raised LDL or triglycerides, or low HDL, consider taking 500–1,000mg of niacin twice a day.
- If you are at risk of atherosclerosis, for example if you are suffering from angina, experiment with a trial period of three months also taking 6g of vitamin C and 3g of lysine daily, in two or three doses. Lysine is better absorbed away from food.
- You can combine niacin with vitamin C and lysine.

Chapter 22 helps you build your own supplement programme.

CHAPTER 12

Antioxidant Protection – Why You Need More than Vitamin E

ack in the 1990s there was a simple theory: oxidants, which are produced from 'burning' glucose for energy within the cells – and are also produced from barbecued meat, chips, cigarettes, and other things – could damage the arteries, cholesterol and the heart; therefore the answer to reducing your risk of heart disease was to take high amounts of *anti*oxidants. The antioxidant 'heroes' were vitamins C and E, the latter being especially important because, unlike vitamin C, which is a water-based antioxidant, vitamin E actually protects fats from damage.

Studies had found, and continue to find, that the higher your intake, or blood levels, of antioxidants the lower your risk. In one study, published in 1993 in the *New England Journal of Medicine*, it was found that 87,200 nurses in the highest fifth of vitamin E intake (equivalent to a daily intake of 100iu (67mg) of vitamin E for more than two years) had a 40 per cent lower risk than those in the lowest fifth of intake.[100] The same was also found to be true in men.[101] Another study involving 11,178 people aged 67–105 found that those supplementing vitamin E over a ten-year period had a 33 per cent reduced risk of death from all causes, and a 47 per cent reduction in death from a heart attack.[102] The same is also true for vitamin C. A UK-based study of 20,000 people published in 2011 in the *American*

Heart Journal reports that the risk of heart failure was cut by 38 per cent for those people who were in the highest quarter of vitamin C blood (plasma) levels.[103] Having a high intake of vitamins E and C from fruits, vegetables, nuts, seeds, seafood and supplements appears to be very good news.

Vitamin E – does it work?

Clinical trials confirmed that giving vitamin E could cut your risk; for example, a large-scale controlled trial on vitamin E, carried out by Professor Morris Brown and colleagues at Cambridge University in 1996, showed a 75 per cent decrease in heart attacks in a group of 2,000 patients with heart disease taking vitamin E, compared to those on a placebo.[104] These results are approximately three times better than the protection offered by aspirin. 'Vitamin E reduced the risk of heart attack by a massive 75 per cent', said Professor Brown, the lead author.

However, a series of trials since 2002 have failed to show any protective effect, and a couple have hinted at a slightly increased risk in cardiovascular patients given vitamin E. Why the difference? One big contender was that the vast majority of people in these trials were taking statins, and statins interfere with vitamin E's antioxidant potential.

How antioxidants work

Antioxidants are team players. What happens in the body is something like a game of 'pass the parcel' except that the 'parcel' in this case is an oxidant – or an oxidising radical, as it is known – and it's more like a hot potato than a parcel. The antioxidant is like an oven glove, which stops the oxidant from burning you, but the antioxidant becomes hot in the process and itself becomes an oxidant. Ultimately, if you've got enough of the right nutrients you'll quench the oxidant and reload the antioxidants to go back to work ready to disarm the next oxidant. You can see a typical sequence in the figure below.

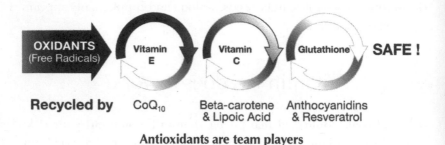

Antioxidants are team players

Statins inhibit vitamin E's antioxidant action

As we saw in Chapter 6 one of the unfortunate side effects of statin drugs is that they knock out CoQ_{10}, and without CoQ_{10} vitamin E cannot properly protect you because it becomes an oxidant.[105] I am not alone in pointing this out. In 2011 a review in a cardiovascular journal stated:

> We analyzed four E vitamin trials from a critical point of view. The protocols neglected an essential fact: that the impact of some confounding factors, such as concomitant use of statins, aspirin and other drugs, might have led to bias and an inappropriate interpretation of the data. The cardiovascular protective and preventive effects of statins and aspirin might have reduced or abolished the possibility of observing a difference in the number of events between the vitamin and placebo groups for the clinical endpoints.'[106]

Of course, the earlier trials happened before the advent of statins. (The use of aspirin, as discussed in Chapter 6, appears to interfere with the effects of B vitamins taken to lower homocysteine.) I approached the authors of these trials and asked if they were intending to analyse the difference between the patients in the trial who were on vitamin E, but not on statins (a small percentage). The answer was either 'no', or I got no response. The results of this kind of negative study get hammered home by including them in reviews and meta-analyses until the general public and doctors are bludgeoned into the belief that vitamin E is dead and buried.

This contentious issue could easily be resolved, either by giving vitamin E to heart patients who were not taking statins, or by at least measuring the antioxidant effect of vitamin E with a blood test. That way you'd know if the drugs were stopping vitamin E from working as an antioxidant, or if vitamin E just wasn't working. These kinds of trials have yet to be done, so we will have to wait and see.

Provided you are not on a statin and you include CoQ_{10} in your supplement programme, though, the chances are that vitamin E is still protective, even after a heart attack, at levels up to 400mg. You should, however, speak to your doctor before taking more than 300mg of vitamin E if you are on blood-thinning medication, as vitamin E does have a blood-thinning effect.[107] (See page 65 for more on combining cardiovascular drugs with natural blood thinners.)

What about vitamin C?

As we saw in Chapter 11, vitamin C does just about everything you could want: it lowers LDL cholesterol, reduces arterial thickening (atherosclerosis), reduces inflammation and cuts your risk of heart attack and stroke. Also, the more you take in the lower your blood pressure becomes.[108] One double-blind study gave 1,000mg of vitamin C or a placebo to participants and found a significant reduction in the systolic blood pressure, but not the diastolic. The team, at the Alcorn State University in Mississippi, concluded that 'vitamin C supplementation may have therapeutic value in human hypertensive disease'.[109] Another study, from 1992, gave 2g to participants and found a 10-point drop in systolic blood pressure in only 30 days.[110]

A meta-analysis of twenty-nine trials confirms that a mere 50mg of vitamin C a day lowers blood pressure by five points in eight weeks.[111] It's also protective. A review of studies on antioxidant intake from 2004 found that those people who supplemented in excess of 700mg of vitamin C a day cut their risk of developing cardiovascular disease by a quarter.[112]

Another potential benefit of vitamin C is that it keeps calcium in solution. Calcium deposition in atheromas (arterial deposits) plays a significant role in arterial blockage. In fact, a test that measures how much calcium you have in your arteries, called CAC (short for coronary artery calcium), is a very good predictor of the degree of atherosclerosis.[113]

One treatment for putting calcium in solution is chelation therapy, which uses a chelating agent (from the word *chela* in Greek, which means 'claw') – an infusion of ethylenediaminetetraacetic acid (EDTA) – to break down arterial deposits. Vitamin C also does this, so having a high circulating amount of vitamin C might help to prevent arterial deposits of calcium.

Supplementing both vitamins C and E was found in a study from 1996 to cut the overall risk of death by 42 per cent and the risk of death from a heart attack by 52 per cent.[114]

The big lesson in the last decade is that it isn't just about vitamins C and E, nor is it as simple as 'oxidants cause diseases and antioxidants prevent them'. The body actually uses oxidation as a positive process in a number of instances, including fighting cancer and infections. What we are learning is that antioxidants support each other and that you can't just give one or two; you need the whole family.

Meet the antioxidant family

As you can see in the illustration on page 124, we all need CoQ_{10} to help recycle vitamin E, and beta-carotene and alpha lipoic acid to recycle vitamin C, as well as anthocyanidins (the blue stuff in berries and red grapes) to recycle glutathione, which is a potent antioxidant also made from the amino acid NAC. Glutathione is also dependent on the mineral selenium. Even this is a vast oversimplification. There are many types of 'vitamin E' called tocopherols and tocotrienols and many other potent antioxidants and anti-inflammatory nutrients found in food that can help protect you.

The idea of just giving one antioxidant is really buying into the drug model, rather than understanding the body as a complex adaptive organism. Hence, there is more logic to giving combinations of antioxidants than putting all your expectations on one player.

An example of this is a study in Israel that gave either a combination of vitamin C (500mg), vitamin E (200iu), selenium (100mcg) and CoQ_{10} (60mg) or placebo to patients with multiple risk factors for heart disease.[115] After six months those on the supplements had clear improvements in arterial elasticity, a reduction in glycosylated haemoglobin (see Chapter 8) and a healthy increase in HDL.

CoQ_{10} and your heart

One major player in the antioxidant family is co-enzyme Q_{10} (abbreviated to CoQ_{10}). It is an antioxidant made by the body that helps heart and all muscle cells to become more efficient. After the age of 40, your levels of this enzyme begin to gradually decline, falling off precipitously in your eighties – a drop that comes at just the time when congestive heart failure becomes more common. CoQ_{10}'s positive effects on heart health are documented in over 100 clinical studies.[116] It is, however, very hard to get enough of it from food (see 'Foods rich in CoQ_{10}' below). Oily fish, nuts and seeds are the best food sources.

Foods rich in CoQ_{10}
(milligrams per 100g)

Food	Amount	Food	Amount
Meat		**Beans**	
Beef	3.1	Green beans	0.58
Pork	2.4–4.1	Soya beans	0.29
Chicken	2.1	Aduki beans	0.22

Fish		Nuts and seeds	
Sardines	6.4	Peanuts	2.7
Mackerel	4.3	Sesame seeds	2.3
Flat fish	0.5	Walnuts	1.9

Grains		Vegetables	
Rice bran	0.54	Spinach	1
Rice	-	Broccoli	0.8
Wheatgerm	0.35	Peppers	0.3
Wheatflour	-	Carrots	0.2
Millet	0.15		
Buckwheat	0.13	Oils	
		Soya oil	9.2

CoQ$_{10}$ – essential for supporting healthy heart function

There are many studies showing that CoQ$_{10}$ has a positive effect on heart and artery health.[117] In over 20 properly controlled studies published in the last two years, CoQ$_{10}$ has repeatedly demonstrated a remarkable ability to improve heart function, and it is now the treatment of choice in Japan for congestive heart failure, angina and high blood pressure, especially among older people.

CoQ$_{10}$, at a daily dose of 90mg, has also been shown to reduce oxidation damage in the arteries, thereby protecting fats in the blood, such as LDL cholesterol, from becoming damaged and contributing to arterial blockages.[118] Together with carnitine, it helps the heart to function more efficiently (more on this in Chapter 19).

A six-year study of people with congestive heart failure, conducted at the University of Texas in the US, found that 75 per cent of the group on CoQ$_{10}$ survived for three years whereas only 25 per cent of a similar group on conventional medication lived as long.[119]

Angina is usually caused by blockages in the tiny arteries that feed the heart muscle cells with oxygen; sufferers feel severe pain in the heart area when exerting themselves. In one study from 1986 at Hamamatsu University in Japan, angina patients treated with CoQ$_{10}$ were able to increase their tolerance to exercise and had less frequent angina attacks.[120] After only four weeks on CoQ_{10}, the patients were able to halve the other medication they were taking. In another trial, from 2004, researchers demonstrated that CoQ_{10} treatment increased the capacity of elderly people to sustain a cardiac workload by 28 per cent.[121]

As well as enhancing antioxidation and protecting nitric oxide (NO), CoQ_{10} also promotes vasodilation in the arteries of those with coronary artery disease, which is exactly what you need to reverse arterial damage and keep the pressure down.[122] It also improves heart function within four weeks in those with heart failure, when given at a dosage of 100mg a day, without any side effects,[123] and it protects heart muscle tissue from the stress of cardiac surgery.[124] In people with quite advanced atherosclerosis it reduces risk and, in those on statins, it reduces fatigue.[125]

If you have heart failure, significant atherosclerosis or angina, CoQ_{10}, at a dose of 90–120mg a day, is a must. It's also essential if you are on statins.

You need CoQ_{10} if you are taking statins

As we saw in Chapter 6, statin drugs inhibit the body's production of CoQ_{10} and therefore impact on energy production by muscle cells, contributing to muscular pain. Research in the US has shown that a high-dose supplement of CoQ_{10} can reverse muscle pains. Fifty patients who had been on statins for two years were taken off the drug because they were complaining of muscle pains and other side effects. Giving them CoQ_{10} dramatically improved their symptoms.[126] Like others, the scientist in this trial commented that statin-related side effects were much more common than the big studies show. He also found that taking the patients off statins didn't make their blocked-up arteries any worse. As mentioned earlier, a warning on statin packets is now mandatory in Canada (but not in the UK or Ireland), saying that the induced CoQ_{10} deficiency reduction 'could lead to impaired cardiac function in patients with borderline congestive heart failure'.

As I stated previously, there are many studies showing that CoQ_{10} has a positive effect on heart and artery health.[127] I recommend taking 30–60mg a day for prevention, and 90–120mg a day if you have cardiovascular disease, together with 200mg of vitamin E. CoQ_{10} in the reduced form known as ubiquinone is most readily absorbed into the blood. It's especially important to supplement this form if you already have heart disease, as it most readily increases your blood levels.[128]

Glutathione (the master antioxidant), NAC and selenium

Possibly the single most important antioxidant in the body is glutathione. If you have lots inside your cells you are more likely to be fighting fit. It is made from the amino acid N-acetyl cysteine, or NAC for short. This is a sulphur-containing amino acid found in eggs, onions, garlic and fish (unsurprisingly perhaps, the supplements smell decidedly eggy). Many people prefer to supplement NAC, however, because glutathione is such a potent detoxifier that it is often used up on its journey into your gut to the cells. Hence the precursor, NAC, may result in increasing cellular levels of glutathione better than giving glutathione itself. However, if glutathione is given with anthocyanadins – red/blue berry extracts – these recycle sacrificed glutathione and therefore are just as good as NAC. So, providing the building material, NAC, which allows the cells to make more glutathione, makes sense. Glutathione can, however, be 'reloaded' after disarming an oxidant by the anthocyanidins found in berry extracts. So supplementing or eating both together provides extra benefit. Glutathione does most of its good work by being converted into a critical antioxidant enzyme called glutathione peroxidase.

Logic, and plenty of circumstantial evidence, suggests that increasing your glutathione levels means decreasing your cardiovascular risk.[129] NAC also stops platelets in the blood from clumping together, it increases glutathione levels in the platelets, which gives them more protection from oxidants, and it increases nitric oxide, which is a powerful anti-clotting factor.[130]

Glutathione peroxidase is dependent on selenium, an essential mineral found in seafood and some nuts and seeds. Other than seafood, the level of selenium present in food will depend very much on the level of selenium in the soil where it grew. Although many books will say that, for example, Brazil nuts are high in selenium, some contain virtually none. Selenium is a mineral that is well worth supplementing, because the majority of adults fail to achieve the basic RDA. Around half of all adult women and older girls, and a fifth of men and older boys, in the UK have intakes of selenium that are at a 'gross deficiency level', according to the UK Food Standards Agency's annual food survey.[131]

If you increase your intake of oily fish, which is also high in omega-3s, you'll be getting more selenium. Some people are concerned that such fish might also be high in mercury. Selenium also protects against mercury's harmful effects, so all in all the overall effect of eating oily fish for cardiovascular health is beneficial.[132]

The other antioxidant you may have noticed in the illustration 'Antioxidants are team players' on page 124 is alpha-lipoic acid. Although research is in its infancy, there is evidence in animal studies that alpha-lipoic acid helps to restore blood flow to the heart after a heart attack. Current research suggests that alpha-lipoic acid plays a protective role against heart attack injury because of its antioxidant and anti-inflammatory effects.[133]

The other family members, including beta-carotene in orange foods, and anthocyanidins and resveratrol in blue/red foods, have all sorts of potential benefits for cardiovascular health.

All-round antioxidant protection

It is highly likely that the best way to get all-round antioxidant protection is to eat a diet especially rich in natural antioxidants and to take a multi-antioxidant supplement. The best protective foods are shown on pages 132–3. These contain not only vitamins A, C and E but many other key antioxidant nutrients such as anthocyanidins, glutathione or cysteine, selenium and more. So the golden rule is to eat at least five to six servings of fresh fruit and vegetables a day and to make sure your diet is rich in naturally multicoloured foods. Green, red, yellow and blue foods such as broccoli, strawberries, avocados and blueberries all provide a varied and rich supply of antioxidants to fight off the oxidants that invade your arteries and damage blood fats. Simply going for an antioxidant-rich 'rainbow' diet has been shown to cut stroke risk by a quarter.[134] Many of these antioxidant foods are also natural anti-inflammatories offering further protection towards keeping your arteries healthy (see Chapter 14).

Measuring a food's ORAC score to find the super-antioxidants

The way to know the antioxidant power of a food is to measure its ORAC (oxygen radical absorbency capacity) potential. This is an objective measure of how good a food is at dealing with the oxidant 'exhaust fumes' of life.

6,000 ORACs a day keeps your heart healthy

The chart below shows the ORACs of 20 different foods that you can incorporate easily into your daily diet. Each serving contains approximately 2,000 units. Just choose at least three of these daily to hit your anti-ageing score of 6,000.

- ⅓ tsp ground cinnamon
- ½ tsp dried oregano
- ½ tsp ground turmeric
- 1 heaped tsp mustard
- ⅕ cup blueberries
- Half a pear, grapefruit or plum
- ½ cup blackcurrants, berries, raspberries or strawberries

- 7 walnut halves
- 8 pecan halves
- ¼ cup pistachio nuts
- ½ cup cooked lentils
- 1 cup cooked kidney beans
- ⅓ medium avocado
- ½ cup red cabbage
- ½ cup cherries or a shot of Cherry Active concentrate

- 2 cups broccoli florets
- 1 medium artichoke or 8 spears of asparagus
- ⅓ medium (150ml) glass red wine
- An orange or apple
- 4 pieces of dark chocolate (70% cocoa solids)

Source: Oxygen Radical Absorbance Capacity of Selected Foods – 2007, US Department of Agriculture

How to get the most antioxidants

Generally speaking, where you find the most colour and flavour you will also find the highest antioxidant levels. The reds, yellows and oranges of tomatoes and carrots, for example, are caused by the presence of beta-carotene. Artichoke, broccoli and avocado have the highest ratings of all the vegetables, while berries, cherries and citrus fruit are the best fruits, so aim for five or more servings daily of a range of fruits and vegetables to keep your intake high.

Foods that have the highest levels are those with the deepest colour, such as blueberries, strawberries, raspberries, cinnamon, turmeric and mustard. One cup of blueberries will provide 9,697 units. You would need to eat 11 bananas to get the same benefit!

The cherry on the top

One of the simplest and easiest ways to achieve 6,000 ORACs is to have a daily shot of a Montmorency cherry concentrate, called Cherry Active, diluted with water. This measures 8,260 on the ORAC scale, which is the equivalent of around 23 portions of regular fruit and vegetables! Although other juices – from acai to pomegranate – claim high ORAC scores, this one tops the lot.

Not just any 'five a day'

The number of portions of fruit and vegetables you need per day really does depend on which ones you choose, as you can see in the menus for two days below. Both days have five portions selected, but Day 2's selection is 8,000 ORACs more than that for Day 1.

DAY 1		DAY 2	
Fruit/vegetable portion	ORAC	Fruit/vegetable portion	ORAC
⅛ large cantaloupe melon	315	Half a pear	2,617
Kiwi fruit	802	Half a cup of strawberries	2,683
1 medium carrot, raw	406	Half an avocado	2,899
Half a cup green peas, frozen	432	1 cup broccoli, raw	1,226
1 cup spinach, raw	455	4 spears asparagus, boiled	986
Total score	2,410	Total score	10,411

Chocolate is good for you

Chocolate, at least the raw stuff, without sugar and milk, is also good for you. Eating antioxidant-rich cocoa products may improve blood pressure and boost levels of good cholesterol, according to a meta-analysis of studies.[135] Consumption of flavonoid-rich cocoa was associated with an average decrease in systolic blood pressure of about 1.6 mmHg, say researchers from Harvard School of Public Health. Writing in the *Journal of Nutrition*, the scientists also report a significant increase in levels of HDL cholesterol following consumption of antioxidant-rich cocoa. In addition, cocoa consumption produced a 1.5 per cent increase in so-called flow-mediated dilation, a measure of a blood vessel's healthy ability to relax. The maximum effects were observed for a flavonoid dose of 500mg/d from cocoa.

The reason for the beneficial effect of chocolate is that it is very rich in two potent antioxidant flavonoids called gallic acid and epicatechin. In fact, chocolate contains roughly twice as much as red wine and four times as much as green tea, which both boast high levels. A group of researchers at Cornell University, led by Chang Lee, found 611mg of gallic acid equivalents (GAE) and 564mg of the flavonoid epicatechin equivalents (ECE) in a single serving of cocoa. Examining a glass of red wine, the researchers found 340mg of GAE and 163mg of ECE. In a cup of green tea, they found 165mg of GAE and 47mg of ECE.[136] So, chocolate came out trumps for these antioxidants.

It must be dark chocolate, however, according to another intriguing experiment,[137] because dark chocolate contains about twice the amount of flavonoids as milk chocolate. In this double-blind experiment 12 healthy volunteers were given either 100g (3½oz) of plain chocolate or 200g (7oz) of milk chocolate. Some were also given 200ml (7fl oz/⅓ pint) of milk to drink, in addition to the dark chocolate. 'Those volunteers who had dark chocolate had a 20 per cent increase in antioxidants in their plasma,' says Alan Crozier, one of the team at the University of Glasgow. 'But those who had milk chocolate, or milk with their dark chocolate, showed no increase in epicatechin plasma levels.' Four hours after eating the chocolate, all the volunteers' blood antioxidant levels had returned to normal. To gain the maximum potential benefits from chocolate, Crozier suggests it may be advisable to refrain from milk products during the four hours after you eat chocolate. Presumably the epicatechins are binding to the milk proteins. Dairy products may inhibit the body's absorption of flavonoids from other foods as well.

Reduce your exposure to oxidants

The flip side to the antioxidant equation is to reduce your exposure to oxidants. The more carbs you eat the more oxidants you make, but you also take in oxidants from eating or breathing the 'exhaust fumes' of anything burnt, be it barbecued meat, crispy bacon and cheese, exhaust fumes and, most of all, cigarettes: each puff introduces you to a trillion oxidants.

Smoking triggers off cell damage, starves healthy cells of oxygen, thickens the blood and raises your blood pressure. Of the deaths caused by smoking, twice as many are due to diseases of the heart and arteries than are due to lung cancer. The less you smoke the better – but best of all, stop smoking. It is also a potent stimulant and induces a state of stress in the body which, as you saw in Chapter 9, is a significant contributor to heart disease. This is essential advice for anyone with heart disease. If you want help doing so, read my book *How to Quit Without Feeling S**t*.

Summary

To maximise your heart health, make these your daily habits:

- Avoid – or minimise your intake of – deep-fried food or burnt, brown or crispy meat.
- Don't smoke, and minimise your exposure to smoke and pollution.
- Eat multicoloured foods with strong red, blue, orange, yellow and green colours.
- Use oregano, cinnamon, mustard and turmeric liberally in cooking.
- Have a good-quality glass of red wine.
- Eat dairy-free dark chocolate on its own, away from milk.
- Supplement additional vitamin A, beta-carotene, vitamin C, vitamin E, CoQ_{10}, glutathione or NAC, alpha-lipoic acid and selenium (see Chapter 22 for recommended doses). You can get most of these in a single antioxidant complex.
- If you are on statins, supplement at least 90mg of CoQ_{10} a day (but speak to your doctor first if you are taking blood thinners).

Chapter 22 helps you build your own supplement programme.

CHAPTER 13

Increase Magnesium and Potassium and Reduce Sodium

Maria, an elderly lady, had angina. Although there was evidence of atherosclerosis in her coronary arteries, this didn't fully explain her angina attacks, which didn't conform to the usual pattern of pain on exertion or after eating a large or high-fat meal. Her doctors advised a coronary bypass operation, to bypass partially blocked arteries. As they were performing the operation they witnessed something unusual and life threatening. One of her coronary arteries went into complete spasm, becoming stiff and hard. They were witnessing a coronary artery spasm, now known to occur when there is severe magnesium deficiency. This is the likely explanation for a small number of heart attack victims who, on autopsy, are not found to have complete arterial blockage. It may also be a factor in heart failure since magnesium is vital for the proper firing of the heart muscle.

This story explains the known connection between having a low level of magnesium and a high risk of heart disease. In fact, heart attack victims tend to have 30 per cent less magnesium and more calcium than normal.[138] Cardiovascular risk is also higher in parts of the world where either the dietary intake or intake of magnesium from water is low. The risk of heart disease is lower in hard water areas, where the water provides more calcium and magnesium. Modern diets are deficient in magnesium, which is found richly in vegetables, nuts, seeds and whole foods but in low amounts in refined foods, meat and dairy produce. The average diet only provides 272mg, compared to the RDA of 300mg or the optimal intake of 500mg a day. That means half the population fall short on magnesium.

Relax with magnesium

One of the main roles of magnesium, together with calcium, is to control the contraction and relaxation of muscles. Both calcium and magnesium atoms can hold an electrical charge. Their balance inside and outside a muscle cell determines whether the muscle cell will contract or relax. Arteries contain a layer of muscle, which led Professors Burton and Bella Altura, a husband and wife team from State University of New York's Health Science Center, to wonder whether a deficiency in magnesium could cause an artery to spasm, reducing or cutting off the blood supply. Their research,[139] which spanned three decades, proved conclusively that removing magnesium from the environment of blood vessels made them go into spasm, potentially reducing the diameter of an artery to one third, as shown below.

If a person's arteries were already narrowed due to atherosclerosis, such a level of magnesium reduction could initiate a heart attack

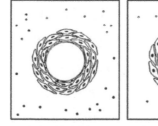 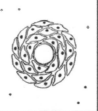 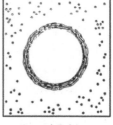

| Normal Calcium and Magnesium | Normal Calcium and low Magnesium | Normal Calcium and high Magnesium |

How magnesium constricts arteries

or stroke. Their research also added a new, inexpensive and harmless therapy for cardiovascular disease: the essential mineral magnesium. A recent meta-analysis of seven studies involving a quarter of a million people found that increasing your intake of magnesium by 100mg a day reduces stroke risk by 9 per cent.[140] This is easily achieved with a serving of greens and seeds a day, or by supplementation. I recommend both.

Magnesium lowers blood pressure

Increasing magnesium intake, especially for those with borderline deficiency, has an immediate effect on lowering blood pressure. As long ago as 1977, researchers from Georgetown University demonstrated an 11 per cent decrease in blood pressure by giving magnesium to those with hypertension.[141] Since then, the relaxing effects of magnesium on the arteries, which also helps reduce anxiety and insomnia, has been well established by numerous research groups.[142,143] What's more, people with high blood pressure do frequently show lower levels of magnesium than those with normal blood pressure. Your health-care practitioner can measure your magnesium status, which is best done by looking at your red blood cell magnesium level.

So, ensuring optimal magnesium intake not only protects you from the risk of high blood pressure but also, for those at cardiovascular risk, reduces the risk of a heart attack. Giving magnesium, usually by injection, during a heart attack also helps stabilise the heart and dramatically reduces the risk of death.

Although much of the research into magnesium's protective effects has focused on its relaxing role in arteries, there is growing evidence that magnesium can also reduce your cholesterol and triglyceride level[144] and that it has an anti-inflammatory effect.[145] Having a low level of magnesium may be as great a risk of cardiovascular disease as having a high cholesterol level, yet it is rarely checked.

Cut back on sodium and increase potassium

The other mineral that reduces blood pressure is potassium; it is found mainly in fruits and vegetables, which are also high in magnesium. Sodium (salt) tightens up the vessel wall, so cutting back is part of official advice and it has been shown to lower blood pressure.[146] According to one study in the *British Medical Journal* eating less salt could cut cardiovascular disease risk by a quarter and fatal heart disease by a fifth.[147] In this study, participants reduced their salt intake by about a third, from 10g to 7g. Over the following 10–15 years their risk of dying from cardiovascular disease went down by 20 per cent; however, just how big an effect is achieved by simply cutting down on salt is still a bone of contention. One review of seven studies found no convincing evidence of a reduced risk,[148] whereas another review of 13 such studies, incorporating 177,000 patients, found that a high-salt diet increased the risk of stroke by 23 per cent.[149]

Part of the Heart-friendly Diet in Part 4 is the recommendation not to add salt to foods as a general rule and to stay away from salted foods.

You'll get the best blood pressure-lowering effects by doing all three – increasing magnesium and potassium, and reducing sodium.[150] The Heart-friendly Diet in Part 4 achieves this, although it is also worth supplementing extra magnesium if you have high blood pressure or a history of heart disease. Potassium is so abundant in vegetables and fruit that you'll get a much bigger effect by eating these rather than taking supplements.

The other benefits of magnesium

Magnesium has many other benefits besides controlling blood pressure. It helps to relax the muscles and mind, promoting better sleep. Diabetics almost always have low levels, as magnesium helps to stabilise blood sugar levels. It's also needed for hormonal balance and it reduces water retention, breast tenderness in PMS as well as cramping and period pains. It may also help menopausal symptoms. If any of these conditions apply to you, you may get extra benefit from increasing your intake of magnesium.

Are you getting enough magnesium?

The worst diet, from the point of view of both heart disease and low magnesium, is one that is high in meat, milk, refined foods and sugar. Not only is such a diet deficient in magnesium but it's also high in calcium. The body needs the right balance of these two 'push-me-pull-you' minerals, which control both nerve and muscle function. Too much calcium in relation to magnesium can cause muscle cramping, irregular heartbeat, high blood pressure, nervousness, irritability and insomnia. Coffee and alcohol also deplete magnesium, as do diuretic drugs. Most people eat about 270mg but need closer to 500mg.

Alternatively, eating a diet rich in vegetables, fruit, nuts and seeds provides more than enough magnesium and calcium, plus potassium, and very little sodium. This is how our ancestors got their calcium. After all, they weren't milking buffaloes! The best sources of magnesium are vegetables, especially greens, and nuts and seeds. The best seeds are pumpkin and chia, followed by sunflower and sesame, while the best nuts are almonds and cashews. Half a cup of pumpkin seeds provides 370mg of magnesium, the ideal daily intake being between 300 and 500mg. Another great food for magnesium is wheatgerm. A spoonful of wheatgerm and ground pumpkin seeds added to your morning cereal ensures added protection against high blood pressure.

Summary

To ensure you have enough magnesium and potassium:

- Make a conscious effort to eat two servings of greens and a small handful of raw nuts or seeds a day. This can increase your intake to 350mg.

- Also supplement 150mg magnesium a day just for prevention. If you have heart disease double this to 300mg. A good multivitamin can provide 150mg (check yours – many have less than 10mg), which is enough for most people. To achieve 300mg a day you'll need to supplement an extra 150mg on top of a good multivitamin–mineral, perhaps with other bone-building nutrients such as calcium, vitamin D and zinc. The perfect ratio is about 2:3 – for example 300mg of magnesium: 450mg of calcium. It works with calcium to control nerve and muscle function, so never supplement calcium without magnesium.
- Also, cut back on coffee and alcohol, which deplete magnesium. (You'll find more on this in Chapter 16.)

Chapter 22 helps you build your own supplement programme.

CHAPTER 14

Are Your Arteries Inflamed?

Every aspect of heart disease, from high blood pressure to arterial and heart damage, involves inflammation. If you could see it, it would look like redness and swelling. If you could feel it, it would be painful. In a state of inflammation the body makes all sorts of pain-producing and inflammatory chemicals with strange-sounding names (CRP, IL-6, TNF alpha, to name a few). The psychological equivalent of inflammation is stress, anger, anxiety and irritability, which, as we saw in Chapter 9, is also a very important part of the heart disease equation.

A mainstay of modern medicine is to suppress the body's ability to produce inflammatory chemicals. This is probably the main reason why aspirin and statins work, although not that effectively. But this is like putting more oil in an engine that is out of tune: you can squeeze out some more life, but what you really need is to tune up the engine.

As you'll see, many of the key factors already discussed – increasing omega-3s, lowering the GL of your diet, lowering your homocysteine, increasing your intake of antioxidants and reducing your stress level – have the effect of preventing your body going into a state of inflammation. Furthermore, the more overweight, or insulin resistant, you are, the more your system will be switched towards reacting in an inflammatory way. By dealing with these issues you are tackling the root cause, not just suppressing your body's attempt to tell you that you're out of whack by taking a drug.

Every time you eat, your body's immune system checks out the food and, in many cases, induces a state of inflammation. This is going to be even worse if you eat high-GL foods that are full of damaged fat (fats that are oxidised through frying or barbecuing, for example, or trans-fats created from food processing), rather than omega-3 fats, when you are stressed. The stress hormone cortisol not only shuts down digestion but also pushes your system into an inflamed state.

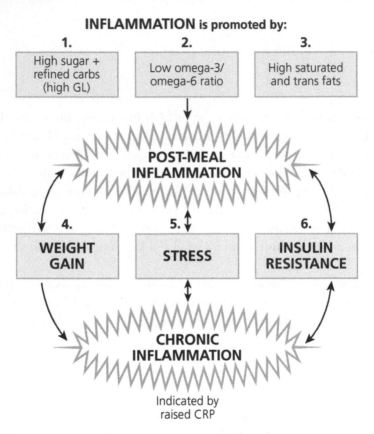

Factors that increase inflammation

How inflamed is your body?

If you had to pick one objective measure of your body's state of inflammation it would be your level of C-reactive protein, abbreviated to CRP. The best way of measuring this is called high-sensitivity

CRP, or hs-CRP for short. This is fast becoming a standard screening test for all sorts of disease processes.

The higher your CRP level the worse off you are likely to be. It is a strong predictor of severity of coronary artery disease.[151] On its own, it's not the best predictor of heart disease but, for a full picture of what's going on, it is certainly worth including. Recent studies are suggesting that having both a raised CRP level and higher levels of CAC (coronary artery calcium – see page 126) is particularly predictive of risk for a coronary event. CRP is another piece of the equation showing you the degree to which inflammation is part of your problem.

Inflammation may also be a critical factor in strokes. In a study of people who had suffered a stroke, CRP proved to be the best indicator of the likelihood of survival, so it is important to reduce your level if it is raised.[152] The ideal level is as low as possible, and certainly below 1mg/dl, although if you do all the right things your level may well be below 0.8mg/dl which is optimal. A level above 2.5mg/dl means roughly double the risk of cardiovascular disease.

What your CRP level means

Low risk	Medium	High	Very high
0.8mg/dl	1.5mg/dl	2.5mg/dl	3mg/dl

Natural anti-inflammatories

Many of the foods that are high in antioxidants are also potent anti-inflammatories. These include curcumin, which is present in turmeric, oleocanthal in olives, hydroxytyrosol in hops, capsaicin in the pepper family, resveratrol in red grapes, and omega-3 fats in fish oils and chia and flax seeds, to name a few.

Which nutrients lower CRP and inflammation?

Omega-3 from both fish and seeds lowers CRP. The more you eat the lower your CRP level and consequent inflammation will be. As your omega-3:6 ratio improves so your CRP reduces.[153] If you have more ALA (alpha-linolenic acid – that's the omega-3 found in seeds such as flax and chia) and less AA (arachidonic acid – that's the fat found in meat and milk) other inflammatory markers will also come down, according to a study of people with blocked coronary arteries.[154]

An increased intake of vitamin E and vitamin C lowers CRP. In a study of people with metabolic syndrome and therefore an increased risk of cardiovascular disease, receiving a combination of vitamin E and C lowered CRP. Giving vitamin E on its own did not.[155]

Other studies confirm the anti-inflammatory effect of the combination of vitamins E and C.[156] It makes sense to take vitamin C, a water-based antioxidant, with vitamin E, a fat-based antioxidant, since they work together to quench oxidants.

Particularly powerful is the combination of omega-3 fish oils with vitamins C and E. This was given to a group of patients after cardiac surgery to see if it would help recovery by decreasing inflammation and oxidation, both of which are critical in the recovery phase after a heart attack or cardiac surgery. The patients were given 1g of vitamin C, 400iu of vitamin E and 2g of omega-3, or the equivalent of two high-potency omega-3 fish oil capsules. CRP levels came down and oxidation reduced, which was measured by looking at levels of glutathione.[157]

Curcumin, the active ingredient in turmeric, has potent anti-inflammatory, antioxidant, anti-thrombotic and cardiovascular protective effects.[158] It may also reduce risk of stroke.[159] In a study where patients with acute coronary heart disease were given either curcumin or a placebo, those on the curcumin had a reduction in their total cholesterol level and their LDL cholesterol level when given 15mg three times a day.

Resveratrol, at a dose of 40mg taken for six weeks by healthy people who were not overweight, has been shown to lower CRP.[160]

The amino acid carnitine, which improves heart function especially if given with CoQ_{10} (more on this in Chapter 19), has been shown to lower CRP at a dose of 1,000mg given for 12 weeks to patients on kidney dialysis.[161]

High-dose zinc, 45mg a day given for six months to 40 healthy elderly people in Detroit, decreased CRP and other inflammatory biomarkers.[162]

The best anti-inflammatory diet

In terms of overall diet, the best for reducing inflammation is a low-GL diet,[163] high in fibre, with oily fish and plenty of fresh fruits and vegetables.[164] A recent review of clinical studies found that increasing dietary fibre reduces CRP[165] so you should aim to eat as much soluble fibre as you can, ideally in the form of oats, barley, rye, aubergine and okra.

Getting your blood sugar under control is critical. When you consume too many high-GI foods or drinks, or you drink too much alcohol, this increases the triglycerides in your blood and this is strongly related to increasing CRP.

All these principles are included in my Heart-friendly Diet in Part 4. A Mediterranean-style diet is certainly heading in the right direction for keeping down inflammation, and it has many other health benefits beyond protecting your heart and arteries.

Although this kind of diet is certainly good for everybody, the extent to which you are likely to benefit from supplementing extra anti-inflammatories depends on whether you are in pain or have a raised CRP level. This is very likely if you already have heart disease, diabetes or metabolic syndrome, or you are significantly overweight with a bit of a 'spare tyre'. In Part 4 I'll show you how to build your own personalised supplement programme based on your particular needs.

Finally, exercising regularly is a great way to lower your level of CRP and inflammation. As you'll see in the next chapter the ideal exercise regime includes both aerobic and resistance exercise, and it is precisely this combination that, when studied in healthy women, has been shown to literally halve CRP levels, from 2mg/dl to 0.8mg/dl, which is an ideal level of CRP.[166]

Summary

Inflammation is a critical process involved in arterial damage. You can measure your level of inflammation with a CRP blood test and reduce it by:

- Following a low-GL, Mediterranean-style diet.
- Eating more fibre.
- Eating oily fish and supplementing omega-3 fish oils.
- Adding turmeric to your meals.
- Eating foods rich in vitamins E and C, and also supplementing them.
- Supplementing resveratrol, carnitine and zinc.
- Exercising, both aerobic and resistance exercise, which is explained in the next chapter.

Chapter 22 helps you build your own supplement programme.

CHAPTER 15

The Exercise Equation

No one would deny that exercise, or at least keeping moderately fit, is a vital part of keeping your heart healthy. After all, anything that gets you physically working strengthens the heart and improves blood flow. There is no doubt that part of the reason for the massive increase in the number of overweight people is that we are becoming less active.[167] And not only does less activity mean fewer calories burnt but it also interferes with the body's appetite mechanisms, rate of metabolism and ability to keep blood glucose, triglycerides and cholesterol levels stable. In other words, some exercise is essential for the body's chemistry to stay 'in tune' as well as for keeping the heart and circulation strong. It may even be as important as your diet.

In an experiment designed to determine which was more important – diet or exercise – Bill Solomon, from the University of Arizona, got some obliging pigs to run around a track, but fed them the average vitamin-deficient diet. Another group ate the pig-equivalent of health food but had no exercise, and a third group had both exercise and good nutrition. If you are wondering how you get a pig to exercise, Solomon built a track and the exercise group were cajoled into their daily jog. Some did it with gay abandon. Others were more resistant, much like some of us! Needless to say, the third group of pigs fared best, proving that exercise and good nutrition together are vital for a healthy heart.

Moderate fitness makes a big difference

Keeping even moderately fit with an active lifestyle makes a big difference to your risk of heart disease. In the massive INTERHEART study (see page 93) regular physical activity accounted for 12 per cent of the risk of heart disease.[168] The fitter you are the lower your risk. To put this into context, a study of 5,314 men between the ages of 65 and 92 found that those who were reasonably fit, compared to the least fit, reduced their risk of death by 38 per cent, whereas those who were most fit reduced their risk of dying by 61 per cent. Those who were unfit and then did something about it cut their risk of premature death by a third.[169]

The combination of keeping physically active and moderate alcohol consumption halves the incidence of having a fatal atherosclerotic heart attack as well as dying from any cause, according to a study of 12,000 Danish adults followed over 20 years, published in the *European Heart Journal*.[170]

Those who engaged in at least moderate exercise had a lower risk of fatal heart attacks and all-cause mortality than people who didn't exercise, and moderate drinkers (meaning 1–14 drinks a week) had lower risks of death than non-drinkers. The combination of the two – physical activity and moderate drinking – appeared even more beneficial, halving the risk of a fatal heart attack.

The many benefits of exercise

If you've been told that you have to exercise to burn calories you've probably done the maths and soon realised it doesn't quite add up. Twenty minutes of jogging equals one American-style chocolate chip cookie, so how motivating is that?

There is so much more going on when you exercise than the calorie equation, however. Exercise is the final puzzle piece in the process of reversing heart disease, metabolic syndrome and losing weight, all of which are often intertwined. Let's take a look at why, and how, it works.

Why you should exercise

If you haven't led a very active life, or you did once but have gradually become more sedentary, that's hardly surprising. Life in the West conspires against exercise. Cars, remote controls, food processors, home-delivery restaurants, home-entertainment centres, escalators, lifts ... every year, there are more gadgets and mod cons that do away with the need to expend energy. Ultimately, all roads lead straight to the sofa and, if you give in, couch-potato syndrome awaits. Unlike eating, most of us are not hard-wired to exercise. In the old days it was something you did to get food. It is, however, a habit you need to cultivate for a number of good reasons. Here are a few of them:

1   **Exercising regularly helps you lose weight** OK, so running a mile a day only burns up 300 calories. But if you do that three days a week for a year, that's 22,000 calories, equivalent to a weight loss of 5kg (11lb)! Also, the number of calories you burn up depends on how fat or fit you are to start with. The fatter and less fit you are, the more benefit you'll derive from small bouts of exercise.

2   **Moderate exercise decreases your appetite** A degree of physical activity is necessary for appetite mechanisms to work properly. Those who do not exercise have exaggerated appetites and hence the pounds gradually creep on. Often you'll find that after a burst of activity you don't actually feel like eating.

3   **Exercise boosts your metabolic rate** According to Professor William McArdle,[171] exercise physiologist at City University, New York, 'Most people can generate metabolic rates that are eight to 10 times above their resting value during sustained cycling, running or swimming. Complementing this increased metabolic rate is the observation that vigorous exercise will raise metabolic rate for up to 15 hours after exercise.' Your metabolic rate is also to do with how quickly the liver breaks down glycogen or fat for fuel. Exercise speeds this process up. Also, if you have eaten more carbs than you need, and the excess is dumped in the liver,

exercising helps you to burn this off before you put it into storage as fat. That's why it is good to go for a stroll after a meal. It helps to stabilise your blood sugar and insulin level and stops you making fat.

4   **Exercise improves insulin sensitivity** Being overweight reduces insulin sensitivity so the risk of developing diabetes is higher. Exercise increases insulin sensitivity, thereby reducing risk. A 24-year study of nearly 6,000 men found that increased physical activity was linked to a reduction in the risk of diabetes, regardless of the level of obesity. It also lowers your glycosylated haemoglobin.

When you exercise, your muscles require glucose, so exercise stimulates the insulin receptors to become more sensitive, reversing insulin resistance. This means that regular exercise helps your blood sugar to become more balanced because insulin starts to work properly.

5   **Exercise promotes the production of growth hormone**, and also testosterone, both of which help to reduce metabolic syndrome. As these hormones go up, the stress hormone cortisol, which is a major promoter of insulin resistance, goes down.

6   **Exercise is a great way to reduce stress** As we learnt in Chapter 9, exercise helps to turn off the stress response.

7   **Exercise reduces your risk of heart disease**, as we saw above, and lowers your cholesterol level and blood pressure.

8   **Exercise reduces inflammation**, lowering your level of CRP, as I explained in the last chapter.

To illustrate the above, an Italian study, published in the *Archives of Internal Medicine*, had a group of 606 diabetics join either a twice-weekly aerobics group, plus receive and act on advice on exercising, or a control group who just received counselling. At the end of a year only those in the exercise group had lowered glycosylated haemoglobin, insulin resistance, blood pressure, cholesterol, waist circumference and body mass index (BMI).[172] Overall, that means less metabolic syndrome. Another similar study, this time in Korea, reported similar benefits in people with metabolic syndrome who followed a combination of diet, exercise and counselling.[173]

In short, exercise offers a huge array of benefits. If you haven't really got into it before, it opens up an undiscovered world of vitality, health – and sheer enjoyment. As your energy returns on my diet you'll soon find you really do gain health and vitality through regular exercise.

Aerobic exercise: long and steady for heart strength

The best kind of exercise to help to burn fat efficiently is aerobic exercise such as brisk walking, jogging, cycling, swimming, aerobic dance, stepping, cross-country skiing, circuit training or any exercise that is long in duration and steady, continuous and of a certain intensity.

Such exercises also tone the body, reduce the risk of osteoporosis, increase muscle tissue and reduce the body fat percentage (high ratios of body fat to lean tissue have been linked to heart disease, diabetes and some cancers). These exercises will strengthen your heart and lungs, reduce your risk of heart disease, help control stress and improve circulation.

Resistance training: building muscle to burn fat

You also need to do some exercise that helps to build more muscle. This is called resistance training, because muscle is built only when you are resisting some force, such as lifting a weight. This kind of exercise actually lowers the harmful stress hormone cortisol. This was confirmed in a study that gave older men a ten-week workout in the gym. Their testosterone levels went up and their cortisol went down.[174]

You may need to get some advice from a fitness instructor to create your own perfect resistance training. On my website www.holforddiet.com you'll find some simple resistance exercises that you can do at home. At the Holford Zest4Life groups we also offer fitness training with a Zest4Fitness programme, designed by former gladiator Kate Stapleton and Olympic athlete Daley Thompson (see Resources). Rather than using gyms the team gets you outdoors and shows you how to use your natural environment to create the perfect mix of both aerobic and resistance training.

If you are recovering from a heart attack or stroke you'll need some professional advice to find the right kind of exercises for you.

How much exercise should you take?

Exercise shouldn't mean a fanatical struggle for some mythical level of fitness. Even raising your basic level of activity, such as a 15-minute walk to the shops and back, makes a big difference. For maximum effect you should also aim to do the two kinds of exercise mentioned above: aerobic exercise that gets you puffing and builds your stamina and a strong heart; and resistance training, which builds more muscle; the muscle, in turn, burns off fat and sugar more effectively and lowers stress hormones. The important thing, however, is to stay within the 'training heart rate zone' for your age – Chapter 23 shows you how to work this out.

What exercise to take and how to do this are also explained more fully in Chapter 23.

CHAPTER 16

What You Drink Makes a Difference

Everyone knows the old clichés that red wine is good for the heart, and that the longevity of the French is due to its benefits. I am not convinced that either of these is true. Firstly, the French are experiencing a substantial increase in all the same health issues – heart disease, diabetes and obesity – as other European countries. Secondly, the evidence, as you'll see, is that a light or moderate amount of alcohol of any kind seems to reduce risk. Thirdly, there is another explanation for the archetypical extended gastronomic lunch, accompanied by a glass of wine, being a heart disease risk reducer, and that is eating when you are not stressed. Also, the era in France that we are talking about, which is now substantially on the wane, also included much more attention to good-quality food, albeit high in fat, which, as we saw in Chapter 4, is a red herring anyway.

Daily drinking, not in excess, reduces heart disease risk

For at least 6,000 years of recorded history, human beings have enjoyed alcohol. Today, it plays a pivotal role in society and even in the economy, with almost 579 million alcoholic drinks consumed each week in the UK. But with plenty of conflicting stories floating around in the media, many people are rightly mystified: is alcohol good for you, or does it harm you? Obviously, in excess it is very bad, causing liver failure, addiction and aggressive behaviour. That we know, but what about that daily glass or two of wine?

There have been over a thousand studies now published on the link between heart disease and alcohol consumption. Remember the INTERHEART study we discussed in Chapter 9 on stress? Alcohol consumption cut the risk of heart attacks and strokes. That finding has been shown in many more studies; for example, a study from Harvard Medical School finds that light-to-moderate alcohol consumption (meaning at least a drink every three to four days and no more than two drinks a day) cuts cardiovascular deaths from either heart attacks or strokes.[175] There's a good review online showing the evidence,[176] for those who want the details.

Alcohol, in moderation, does many things that are good news for arteries. It increases HDL (good) cholesterol, tends to act as an anti-inflammatory, and even lowers blood pressure. Somewhere around three-plus drinks per day this effect is reversed.

This is true for both beer and wine, and seems to relate more to the quantity drunk than the type of drink. Red wine, in particular, may confer additional cardiovascular benefits by virtue of being high in proanthocyanidins, the antioxidants found in grapes and berries, by reducing arterial stiffness. Alcohol itself, however, is an oxidant.

Another potential benefit of alcohol is a mild reduction in platelet aggregation – in other words, it makes your blood thinner. This occurs because alcohol blocks the formation of prostaglandins from essential fats. For the body to make use of essential fats, however, these fats must be converted into their active compounds – a process which is blocked by alcohol. So the combination of being essential-fat deficient and drinking alcohol is not a good idea.

The bone of contention is the dose: does a glass of wine a day confer benefit? Most reviews conclude that there is a clear risk reduction from light or moderate drinking; however, some studies show a link between moderate to heavy alcohol consumption and increased blood pressure and incidence of strokes. Diabetes risk also appears to be lower with light or moderate drinking, but not heavy drinking.

One strong possibility is that alcohol acts as a relaxant, reducing stress hormones, as we saw in Chapter 9. It is also worth bearing in mind another confounding factor: people who enjoy a glass of wine in the evening are often eating better and having a healthier lifestyle, so some of these studies might tell you more about wine drinkers than wine drinking per se.

Alcohol taxes your liver and your gut

Alcohol is certainly not all good news. It is detoxified by the liver, which involves a liver enzyme called alcohol dehydrogenase, but when you consume more alcohol than this enzyme can handle, the liver will instead metabolise the alcohol to chloral hydrate, also known as Mickey Finn drops, which knock you out. Normally, alcohol is metabolised to acetaldehyde by an enzyme called acetaldehyde oxidase and, from there, to harmless chemicals that can be excreted from the body. But if you overload the liver you end up with too much circulating acetaldehyde. This very acidic and toxic substance leads to ketoacidosis – what we commonly refer to as a hangover: namely headache, nausea, mental and physical tiredness, and aching muscles. Acidosis occurs when the blood has become too acid, in this case through the toxic metabolites of alcohol. Acidosis is a cause of premature ageing and osteoporosis and can lead to other disease states. It is a frequently reported finding in excess alcohol consumption. The liver enzyme responsible for detoxifying alcohol depends on a good supply of antioxidant nutrients, especially vitamin C.

There is little question that alcohol acts as an 'anti-nutrient'. Although some forms of alcohol (such as stout or red wine) do deliver a few nutrients, alcohol itself is a potent destroyer of these same nutrients. Beer, for example, provides small amounts of B vitamins from yeast, and good-quality red wines deliver anthocyanidins including resveratrol. It also affects your nutrient intake by disturbing the digestion and absorption of food, and suppressing appetite. Chronic alcohol consumption leads to multiple deficiencies

157

of nutrients, including B vitamins, vitamin C, magnesium and zinc, all of which are important for cardiovascular health.

Alcohol also irritates your intestinal tract, making it more permeable to undigested food particles and increasing the chances of an allergic reaction to substances in both the food and the alcohol. This is why many beer and wine drinkers become allergic to yeast. Wine drinkers may also become sensitive to sulfites, which are added to grapes to control fermentation. Better choices include organic, sulfite-free wines and champagne – the latter of which has the added bonus of being virtually yeast-free, as are spirits.

As well as increasing intestinal permeability, alcohol wreaks havoc on intestinal bacteria. It has been reported to convert gut bacteria into secondary metabolites that increase proliferation of cells in the colon, initiating cancer. It can also be absorbed directly into the mucosal cells that line the digestive tract and then converted into aldehyde, which interferes with DNA repair and promotes tumours. In addition, some alcoholic drinks contain the carcinogen urethrane. Urethrane has been found in bourbon whiskeys, European fruit brandies such as cherry brandy, cream sherries, port, sake and Chinese wine, but not in vodka, gin and most beers. Since both alcohol and aspirin are intestinal irritants, there is good reason to curtail alcohol consumption if you are on a daily aspirin. Many aspirin preparations designed for long-term use are enteric coated to protect the stomach, but the coating must be broken down in the intestines to absorb the drug.

Does alcohol cause weight gain?

One of the potential concerns about alcohol, certainly in excess, is that it encourages abdominal weight gain and the signs of metabolic syndrome. While this is obviously true in frequent beer drinkers, in a survey of over 19,000 non-obese women who drank a light to moderate amount of alcohol, it was found that, when followed up over 13 years, the women appeared to gain less weight and had a lower risk of becoming overweight and obese than non-drinkers.[177] The survey found that those who drank 15g of alcohol a day, which is the equivalent of a glass of wine, a shot of a spirit or 600ml (20fl oz/1 pint) of beer, were almost 30 per cent less likely to become overweight or obese. The most positive association was found with red wine, followed by white. A beneficial effect was also apparent at 30g a day, but not at 40g a day.

From a glycemic-load point of view I'd be cautious about the pint of beer since this represents 20 GLs – but the ideal daily amount for maximum weight loss is 45GLs, and 65GLs for maintenance, if you do not need to lose weight or when your weight has stabilised. On my Heart-friendly Diet I allow 5GLs a day for drinks or desserts, which is the equivalent of 300ml (10fl oz/½ pint) of beer every other day or a low-carb lager every day (or a glass of wine or spirit).

The hard truth about soft drinks

In the past 20 years, much of the insidious increase in sugar in the modern-day diet has come from soft drinks. Also, in recent years, the principal sugar used has switched from glucose or sucrose, derived from sugar cane, to high-fructose corn syrup, derived from mass-produced corn.

What happens to fructose in the body?

Before we even get into what the body does with fructose, it's clear that drinking any sugared juice or fruit juice exposes you to a massive and sudden increase in sugar, both glucose and fructose. In the case of glucose, 80 per cent goes to cells to burn off, provided you are physically active, leaving 20 per cent that goes to the liver. If you are not physically active and excess glucose is ingested, some of this goes into storage as glycogen; the rest turns into fat. Glucose increases insulin, increasing storage of this as fat, in addition to increasing the storage of fat from food. Because fructose isn't burnt for energy in the same way as glucose is – because cells can't run off fructose – the body has to do something with it, and it turns it into fat in the liver, provided again that you are not physically active.

Fructose might not increase insulin levels or promote fat storage in fat tissue from dietary fat in the same way as glucose does; however, every time you have a glass of fruit juice or a fructose-sweetened soft drink, your liver has to work really hard. There is a limit to the liver's capacity to handle fructose.

When stretched to the limit, the fat that your liver has converted from fructose and other sugars spills out into the liver itself. This means that fat is dumped into the liver. At its extreme this creates a condition known as non-alcoholic fatty liver disease (NAFLD). This also stops insulin working in the liver. If you keep drinking these high-fructose drinks, the body has to produce more insulin. A high-GL diet or high sugar consumption is actually the second most common cause of liver failure and it inevitably leads to raised insulin levels and, in due course, insulin resistance. The consumption of soft drinks increases the prevalence of NAFLD and is also associated with a much greater risk of metabolic syndrome, weight gain and obesity.[178]

In addition, both fructose and high glucose are turned into uric acid in the liver, which then promotes gout.[179] Uric acid also switches off nitrous oxide, which keeps your blood pressure low. So, too much fructose is also associated with high blood pressure. But most of the fructose is turned into the bad LDL cholesterol, and is then put into storage as fat. The bottom line is to keep any form of sugar to a minimum. Anything other than a small amount of fructose in a whole fruit, which naturally contains lots of fibre to 'slow release' the sugar, is closer to a toxin than a nutrient and is best avoided or kept to a minimum.

Cafetiere coffee is especially bad for the heart

Coffee is worse for your heart than tea. Coffee beans contain lipids that raise LDL cholesterol. This effect is pronounced in cafetiere coffee, but not filter coffee, where the coffee is filtered through paper. Six cups of cafetiere coffee can raise cholesterol by 10 per cent and most of this is due to an increase in LDL cholesterol.[180] There is also an increase in triglycerides. Researchers have proposed that the effect is due to two compounds called cafestol and kahweol. The same effect is not seen in filter coffee, so that's the way to go.

What about espresso? It actually has less cafestol and kahweol, so it might be better. Roughly four to five espressos equals one cafetiere coffee in this regard. An Italian study on people drinking three espressos a day didn't find any significant change in LDL cholesterol.[181]

However, heart disease isn't all about cholesterol, as you saw in Chapter 4. Stress, partly through abnormal levels of the adrenal hormone cortisol, plays a major role in heart disease risk. Coffee, and any stimulant in excess, increases this stress response and therefore it is advisable to either avoid it completely or have one cup a day or on the odd occasion, but not as a regular daily addiction, knocking back two or more a day. This is especially important if you are already stressed. So, don't use coffee as a daily pick-me-up.

Drink water when you are thirsty

One of the simplest ways to lower blood pressure and promote your health is to drink six to eight glasses of water a day. It helps lower blood pressure without the side effects because a lack of water makes the sodium level inside cells go up, which raises blood pressure.

You can enjoy life and be healthy too

I am convinced that light drinking has more benefits than negatives for heart disease prevention. I am not a drinker as such – I can go weeks without any. Nor am I a teetotaller, so I don't say this with any particular axe to grind.

For my money, there's a big difference between occasional drinking, and drinking more than 2 units or two small glasses of wine every day. I see many clients who have a mild dependency on even such small daily intakes, and others who find it hard to leave a bottle unfinished, knocking back half a bottle every night with their partners. This is in contrast to the French who traditionally would share a bottle between four or more people, having the equivalent of a glass each with the meal, not half a bottle. If a break for a couple of weeks would pose no problem to you, then that indicates a healthy relationship with alcohol.

On the other hand, if you are optimally nourished and have a healthy liver and digestive system, a glass of (preferably organic) wine or beer three times a week, or even every day, is unlikely to impact your health. In the 100% Health Survey we found no significant change in health scores between those having a drink a day and those who had none.

I would, however, stay away from drinking sweetened drinks, and keep your coffee intake to a minimum, meaning one filter coffee a day maximum.

Summary

To reduce your risk of heart disease:

- Drink a small glass of wine or 300ml (10fl oz/½ pint) of beer three times a week, or no more than one every day.
- Avoid all sweetened drinks.
- Drink coffee rarely, one filter coffee a day maximum.
- Drink six to eight glasses of water a day.

PART 3

HEART-FRIENDLY STRATEGIES FOR RAPID RECOVERY

If you've been diagnosed with high cholesterol or high blood pressure or if you are already suffering from the pain of angina, this part gives you a strategy to rapidly reverse your risk and restore your arteries to health. If you've had a heart attack or stroke you'll learn how to maximise your recovery.

CHAPTER 17

How to Lower Your Cholesterol Without Drugs

As you'll have learnt by now, there are many ways to lower cholesterol naturally without resorting to statin drugs that block the body's ability to make it in the first place. The reason why this is a better place to start is, firstly, because it helps you to address the true underlying causes of high cholesterol and, secondly, because cholesterol-lowering drugs have significant side effects.

That being said, everything in this chapter can be done alongside cholesterol-lowering drugs. My one provision is to encourage you to also take CoQ_{10} if you are on statins (see page 129).

The positive changes you can make that have a direct effect on your cholesterol levels are:

- Following a low-GL diet.

- Increasing plant sterols and soluble fibres.

- Increasing omega-3 fats, both in your diet by eating fish and from supplements.

- Supplementing high-dose niacin (B_3), plus a high-strength multivitamin and extra vitamin C and magnesium.

- Reducing your stress level.

- Exercising and losing weight with a low-GL diet – my Heart-friendly Diet.

Putting all these factors together is a winning formula, as can be seen by the experiences of Mike below:

Case Study: Mike

'In mid-April I had my blood checked and found my cholesterol to be 6.5. I do eat really healthily and felt that my condition was due to hereditary cholesterol rather than dietary factors. A friend had reduced theirs through the supplements recommended in your [Patrick Holford's] book, so I thought it was worth a try. Five weeks later I went for a second blood test to find my cholesterol had dropped to 5.1. My GP couldn't believe it! He would not wholeheartedly acknowledge the success, but he didn't knock it either, saying, "Whatever you are taking is working – come back in a year!"'

Another success story is that of Andrew from Dublin.

Case Study: Andrew

Andrew's cholesterol was 8.8mmol/l. He was also gaining weight, feeling tired and stressed, and not sleeping well. He was put on statins and, six months later, it was 8.7. The lack of response, plus side effects, led him to stop.

Andrew attended one of my 100% Health workshops, changed his diet and started taking supplements including high-dose niacin, vitamin C and omega-3. Three weeks later, he had lost 4.5kg (10lb), his energy levels were great, he no longer felt stressed and he was sleeping much better. And his cholesterol level had dropped to a healthy 4.9.

Your ideal cholesterol

Exactly what your cholesterol statistics mean is explained in Chapter 3. The medical profession's obsession with lowering total cholesterol below 5, and some say even lower, is not consistent with the evidence of what really correlates with risk. Previous 'normal' ranges were up to 6mmol/l. Ideally, you should aim for:

- Total cholesterol below 6 and perhaps ideally below 5.2mmol/l.*

- HDL cholesterol above 1.6mmol/l.

- Cholesterol:HDL ratio equal to or less than 3:1.

- Triglycerides below 1mmol/l.

- Triglycerides:HDL equal to or less than 2:1.

This is the Holy Grail, and when you achieve it there is really no need for medication.

*PLEASE NOTE If your cholesterol:HDL ratio is 3 or less – for example, 6:2 – do not be worried if your cholesterol is above 5.

The low-glycemic-load (GL) diet is the key

Official diet advice is that we should eat lots of starchy carbohydrates such as bread, rice and potatoes. But it is exactly these high-glycemic-load foods that raise your blood sugar and cholesterol levels; examples include bread and cakes made from refined flour, which rapidly release glucose into the bloodstream.

As a way of lowering the risk of heart disease, this is far from ideal. Because they make blood sugar levels soar, high-glycemic foods cause more of the fat-storing hormone insulin to be released, as well as boosting production of the stress hormone cortisol. So what happens to the extra glucose sloshing about in the bloodstream? It gets stored as fat, then up goes your triglyceride levels. In time you become insensitive to insulin and thus make more, which pushes your cholesterol level even higher.

The link between high-glycemic foods and dangerous fat levels showed up clearly in a study in 2007 where mice fed a diet of high-glycemic starchy foods developed a potentially deadly condition known as 'fatty liver'; they also had twice the amount of fat in their bodies as those on a low-glycemic diet even though they weighed the same.[1]

Much more effective for maintaining a healthy heart is the Mediterranean diet. It's based on foods that have had little processing, such as fruits, vegetables, pulses and whole grains, and as a result releases glucose much more slowly into the bloodstream. It also encourages you to eat quite a lot of fat, especially olive oil and omega-3.

The low-glycemic element of the diet will reduce your cholesterol levels and it is also an effective way of losing weight. Meanwhile, the healthy fats help to protect the heart. A meta-analysis of weight-loss studies concluded that 'Overweight or obese people lost more weight on a low Glycaemic Load diet and had more improvement in lipid profiles (cholesterol and triglycerides) than those receiving conventional (low fat, low calorie) diets.'[2] Other benefits were greater loss in body fat, reductions in 'bad' LDL cholesterol, and increases in 'good' HDL cholesterol. In Chapter 8 you will have seen lots of examples of studies that have shown highly significant reductions in cholesterol, and increases in HDL, when people follow a low-GL diet.

Exactly how to follow a low-GL diet is explained in Chapter 21. I should point out that this diet is very precise and has a lower GL per day than most of the studies I've referred to. So, if you need to lose weight, you can expect even better results; however, you will not go hungry.

The importance of plant sterols and soluble fibres

Plant sterols are present in pulses, including beans and lentils. The most researched in this respect is soya, which is why many soya products rightly claim that they help to lower cholesterol. There are also plant sterol-enriched margarines, such as Benecol, which makes similar claims. Studies have shown that the regular consumption of 1–3g of plant sterols per day lowers LDL cholesterol by 5–15 per cent. There's also evidence that the more soya you eat the lower your blood pressure will be.[3]

My Heart-friendly Diet, in Chapter 21, purposely includes 2.5g of plant sterols a day, which is the equivalent of 50g of soya – roughly a glass of soya milk or a small serving of tofu, or a small soya burger. Other foods, including nuts such as almonds, and most beans and lentils, also provide plant sterols, so you can use these if soya isn't your cup of tea. You'll see which foods contain the most plant sterols on page 209.

Soluble fibres are found in oats, okra and aubergine. They are in the bran or rough part of oats so you need to eat whole oat flakes or rough oatcakes, or add oat bran to cereals. One of my favourite sources of soluble fibre is chia seeds, as well as flax seeds (also known as linseed), although chia tastes much better than flax. The soluble fibre-rich foods become 'glooky' when water is added because they absorb a lot of water.

Combining plant sterols with soluble fibres is actually more effective in lowering cholesterol than statins (see page 90) according to a study by Professor David Jenkins from the University of Toronto in Canada. 'People interested in lowering their cholesterol should probably acquire a taste for tofu and oatmeal,' he said.

A simple example of putting these principles into action is eating hummus (made from chickpeas) with rough oatcakes, which gives you both plant sterols and soluble fibres.

You can go one step further by adding the super-soluble fibre glucomannan to your daily diet. This extraordinary fibre, from the Japanese konjac plant, has been shown to lower cholesterol in a number of studies.[4] You need about 3–5g for the best effect, which is roughly a teaspoonful, stirred into a large glass of water, taken just before a meal. This lowers the GL of the meal and may be why it lowers your cholesterol. It's also very good if you are prone to constipation.

Ensure you eat omega-3 fats

For decades now, doctors and nutrition experts have been advising us to eat a low-fat diet, both to lose weight and to protect our hearts; however, this advice looks increasingly as if it may be contributing to making the problem worse, because most low-fat foods are higher in carbohydrate.

In fact, we are now eating less fat than ever before; meanwhile levels of obesity are soaring. It's perfectly clear that the amount of fat you eat has very little to do with putting on weight. As for heart disease, higher levels of the right sort of fat – natural and largely unprocessed – protect your heart.

Even saturated fat is not the demon it is made out to be. Just to give one example – although there are many more – nearly 30,000 middle-aged men and women in Sweden were followed for six years and recorded their food intake. The conclusion was that 'Saturated fat showed no relationship with cardiovascular disease in men. Among women cardiovascular mortality showed a downward trend with increasing saturated fat intake.' In other words the more saturated fat they ate the lower their chance of dying from heart disease.

What is far less controversial is that no healthy-heart diet would be complete without omega-3 fats; many studies show that these not only bring down cholesterol but it can also decrease the levels of harmful triglycerides in the blood as well as reduce the inflammation that's linked with heart disease. We discussed all the evidence in detail in Chapter 7. To recap briefly, a review of ten randomised controlled trials showed that fish oils decrease the triglycerides by an average of 29 per cent, lower cholesterol by 12 per cent, lower the bad LDL cholesterol by 32 per cent and increase HDL by 10 per cent.[5]

NICE recommends that all doctors prescribe 1g of fish oil for six months to patients who have had a heart attack. (Then the budget runs out.)

If your budget can stand it, however, my recommendation is to keep going, supplementing 1g of omega-3-rich fish oil daily, and also eating oily fish three times a week. I take, twice a day, an essential omega capsule that gives me 650mg of combined EPA/DPA/DHA. Together with three servings of oily fish (salmon, mackerel, kippers, sardines, herrings, pilchards) a week, that gives me a total weekly omega-3 intake of over 10g, or 1.5g a day. This is equivalent to what you'd get in two high-potency omega-3-rich fish oil capsules. If you have high cholesterol or have recently had a cardiovascular event, I'd recommend a daily high-potency omega-3 fish oil, plus a basic essential omega supplement, as well as the oily fish. Once your cholesterol statistics are back to normal you could drop the extra omega-3-rich fish oil, but keep going with the essential omegas.

An alternative to the omega-3-rich fish oil is high-strength cod liver oil, which is an excellent dietary source of anti-inflammatory vitamins A and D, but do check that it's got enough EPA and DHA. (You want at least 500mg combined.)

The Heart-friendly Diet (in Chapter 21) and exactly what to supplement (in Chapter 22) build in all these recommendations.

The really bad fats you should avoid are the heavily processed ones such as trans-fats found in foods like margarines and industrially produced baked foods. For steam-frying (a healthy way to cook, explained on page 231) use coconut butter, a little butter or olive oil.

Niacin is a must for raising 'good' HDL cholesterol

Despite the relentless medical focus on reducing levels of LDL cholesterol as a cause of heart disease, 40 per cent of all cardiovascular problems happen in people who have low levels of HDL cholesterol. So drug companies have long tried to develop drugs to increase the amount you have.

Unsurprisingly, the drugs also do other things, which means they can also have dangerous side effects. In the case of one called torcetrapib, these side effects included raised blood pressure; a major clinical trial had to be abandoned because there were 50 per cent more deaths in the group taking it than among those only getting a statin.

According to a major review in the *New England Journal of Medicine* of what works, 'the most effective way' is with vitamin B$_3$ (niacin).[6] Niacin also comes out top in a review of the drug trials to raise HDL, which describes the new medications as 'disappointing'.[7] In Chapter 11 we reviewed the evidence for niacin, which becomes effective at doses of 1,000–2,000mg a day. That's a long way off the RDA of 18mg.

Because niacin is a vitamin, and so part of your body's normal functioning, it is highly unlikely to have the dangerous adverse reactions triggered off by a new single-molecule drug. That's also why most doctors never think of using it. A number of studies have shown that it is effective not only in raising HDL by up to 35 per cent but also in reducing LDL by up to 25 per cent. It also reduces levels of two other markers for heart disease: lipoprotein(a) and fibrinogen. By way of comparison, statins raise HDL only by between 2 per cent and 15 per cent. So, why aren't doctors prescribing niacin?

It's a good question. The lack of prescriptions certainly has nothing to do with a lack of research. Medline, the database of research for the US National Institutes of Health, quotes over 40 positive studies from the last five years recommending niacin over statins, or with statins to further improve their cholesterol-lowering effect.[8] I recommend 1,000mg a day to lower raised LDL cholesterol and to raise a low HDL cholesterol.

Niacin side effects

The most obvious side effect of taking fairly high doses of niacin is a blushing effect, which is diminished by taking the vitamin with food, but non-blush or extended-release niacin is now easily available. Other reported side effects include dyspepsia and fluctuations in blood sugar and uric acid levels, although these last two have not been found in recent studies. A randomised controlled trial reports that of 148 diabetic patients, only four discontinued niacin because of inadequate glucose control.[9] Finally, niacin is best taken with high-dose homocysteine-lowering nutrients (see page 237), as there is some evidence that niacin may otherwise slightly raise homocysteine levels. In any event, I'd recommend anyone with cardiovascular concerns to check their homocysteine levels (see Chapter 10).

There was a hint of a concern in one study that the combination of statins plus niacin might slightly increase stroke risk. It's too early to say if this is really an issue, however. In an ideal world it might be better to try niacin plus all these other recommendations first, because you might just find that your cholesterol levels normalise, rendering the need for statins obsolete.

The form of niacin is important. Although the cheapest is pure niacin, this gives a very strong blushing effect for up to half an hour. Most people find that, within a few days, if you take it twice a day, every day the blushing subsides. You can also reduce the blushing by starting with a low dose of 50–100mg per day, then double the dose each week until an effective level of at least 250mg twice a day is reached.

Alternatively, there are prescribable forms of niacin, such as Niaspan, that don't cause blushing. These are available on prescription from your doctor.

There is also a non-blushing form of niacin called inositol hexanicotinate, which is available in health-food stores. Clinical trials haven't been carried out on this form, so it's hard to say whether it works as well. One woman told me she lowered her cholesterol from 10 to 5.1 in 30 days taking this form of niacin. Another form of niacin, niacinamide, doesn't lower cholesterol. It is possible that the blushing effect may be part of the benefit of niacin. In any event, the lowest therapeutic level is 500mg (one tablet) and the highest is 2,000mg.

Increase magnesium

In Chapter 13 you learnt that the mineral magnesium lowers blood pressure by about 10 per cent,[10] as well as reducing cholesterol and triglycerides,[11] thus substantially lowering the risk of death from cardiovascular disease. Unfortunately, a lot of us are deficient in magnesium – the average intake in the UK is 272mg, whereas an ideal intake for cardiovascular protection is in the region of 500mg – and this is especially likely if you have high blood pressure. The richest source of this mineral is dark green vegetables, nuts and seeds, especially pumpkin seeds. These foods are included in your Heart-friendly Diet; however, it is also worth supplementing at least 150mg of magnesium every day, and double this if you do have high blood pressure or cardiovascular disease. A few good-quality multivitamin and mineral supplements will provide 150mg (but most don't), leaving a further 150mg to supplement. A particularly good form of magnesium is magnesium ascorbate, which is bound to vitamin C, effectively killing two birds with one stone, since vitamin C lowers blood pressure and cardiovascular risk.

Put all this together and you have a winning formula for optimum cholesterol and triglyceride levels.

Learn how to handle stress

A major factor, usually overlooked in the conventional approach to heart problems and raised cholesterol, is stress – both physical and psychological. Of course, stress in the form of exercise or a challenging job can be very good for you, but chronic stress can damage your health and your heart. There is no mystery as to how it happens. Bad stress, which can come from poor working conditions, a bullying boss or few friends, has clear and well-understood effects on your hormones – especially adrenalin and insulin – as well as your nervous system. And this in turn has direct and measurable effects on your body chemistry; in fact, it produces many of the familiar heart disease 'risk' factors.

For example, you respond to stress by producing adrenalin, which in turn pushes up blood sugar levels, raises blood pressure and increases both blood-clotting agents and LDL cholesterol. Meanwhile, extra amounts of the stress hormone cortisol encourage the storage of dangerous 'visceral' fat in the abdomen. And visceral fat is strongly connected to metabolic syndrome, which is a big risk factor for diabetes and heart disease.

So a vital part of any regime aimed at a healthy heart and lowering cholesterol naturally involves turning off a damaging stress response. There are plenty of ways to do it, such as exercise, moderate alcohol consumption, watching your football team winning, passing an exam, or organising an enjoyable social evening. Chapters 9 and 24 give more details.

Exercise and lose weight

Losing weight by following my low-GL diet and exercising both also effectively lower cholesterol. An example of this is the small study we did on 21 people (see page 16) who followed the diet for 12 weeks. Their average cholesterol levels dropped by 13 per cent and the HDL fraction increased. Resistance exercise helps to reverse insulin resistance, and aerobic exercise has been shown, in many studies, to lower cholesterol and triglycerides. Combining a low-GL diet and exercise is a winning formula.

Summary

To lower your cholesterol:

- Follow a low-GL diet (see my Heart-friendly Diet in Chapter 21).
- Increase plant sterols and soluble fibres by eating more beans, lentils, nuts, seeds and oats.
- Supplement high-dose niacin (B_3), at least 500mg twice a day, plus a high-strength multivitamin and extra vitamin C (2g or more) and magnesium (at least 300mg).
- Increase omega-3 fats, both in your diet by eating fish and from daily supplements, providing 1,000mg of EPA in total.
- Reduce your stress level (see Chapter 24).
- Exercise daily (see Chapter 23) and lose weight with the low-GL diet.

Chapter 22 helps you build your own supplement programme.

CHAPTER 18

How to Lower High Blood Pressure Naturally

High blood pressure (BP) is one of the top risk factors for heart disease and stroke. It has been linked with 50 per cent of cases of coronary artery disease and 75 per cent of stroke cases and the effects of it kill over 110,000 people in England every year. It's an essential part of every health check and while doctors know that exercise combined with a low-GL, Mediterranean-style diet rich in fruit and vegetables can bring it down, the general view is that such a regime is hard to stick to, so if your level is up, the chances are you will be offered drugs.

In Chapter 2 I explained how blood pressure is read and that the diastolic measurement (the one written underneath, which gives the blood pressure when your heart is at rest) is the more important measurement. A normal reading would be around 120/76mmHg; if your blood pressure is above 140/90, you have hypertension (high blood pressure). Symptoms of hypertension include nosebleeds, tinnitus (ringing in the ears), dizziness and headaches, but you can easily have hypertension without any signs. Some people have low blood pressure (around 90/60). This is not a problem as long as you're healthy.

Drugs will bring high blood pressure down by an average of 5.5mmHg diastolic, but at a cost. They all come with fairly nasty side effects, which is why many people don't stick to taking them; these range from short-term problems like fatigue, muscle weakness and depression to long-term illness including heart disease and a pre-diabetic state with high levels of insulin and blood sugar.

The drugs are available in four main types and their mechanisms range from relaxing the muscles of the blood vessel walls to making you pee more. The latest trend is to market a combination of two different types in one, with the promise of even more effective lowering.

How blood pressure works

If you want to get control of your blood pressure, it helps to have some idea of how the whole system works; that way it's easier to decide on a treatment plan that's going to work for you. Unlike the pipes in your domestic plumbing system, your blood vessels play an active role in speeding up or slowing down your blood circulation. Their muscular walls tense and relax all the time. When you're frightened or exercising, you need them to tense and narrow to pump more blood around the body, but then they should relax. When they stay tense for too long the result is hypertension.

To re-iterate what I pointed out earlier, it's a complex, normally self-regulating system that is partly controlled by the ebb and flow of two pairs of minerals in and out of the cells lining the blood vessel walls. One of these pairs consists of sodium (salt) and potassium: sodium inside the cell pushes the pressure up; potassium inside brings it down. The other pair consists of calcium and magnesium: calcium raises while magnesium lowers.

This explains why you're advised to keep your salt intake down (more sodium raises BP) and why one of the types of drug is a calcium channel blocker (keeping calcium out lowers BP). But it also highlights the way that two halves of the pairs are largely ignored by the conventional approach. As you saw in Chapter 13, getting good amounts of potassium and magnesium through your diet or via a supplement is a sensible starting point for any BP-lowering regime.

Understanding the system also highlights the downside to some of the drug treatments, such as the diuretics, which make you pee a lot. That in turn means there's less liquid in your blood and so the pressure drops. This downside of this is that a lot of minerals and vitamins are washed out in the process, including potassium and magnesium – precisely the ones you need. There are now potassium-sparing diuretics but, typically, they put you at risk of potassium overload! Drinking enough water, however – six to eight glasses a day – helps to lower blood pressure without the side effects, because a lack of water makes the sodium level inside cells go up, which raises blood pressure.

And there are other problems with diuretics. One study of 1,860 men followed over a period of 17 years found that those treated with diuretics were more likely to have a heart attack (23 per cent) than those who weren't. Those who had a heart attack were more likely to have raised glucose levels, putting them in a pre-diabetic state.[12]

This poor performance by diuretics – an old type of drug but still widely used – is unfortunate since, according to one large study known as ALLHAT, they are more effective than the newer drugs, which includes the calcium channel blockers and another type known as ACE (angiotensin-converting enzyme) inhibitors, which counteract the effect of angiotensin, a body chemical that contracts blood vessels.[13]

A low-GL diet is good for healthy blood pressure

So, given drugs' side effects and doubts about their effectiveness in the long term, the non-drug approach certainly seems to make sense as a starting point. It also offers you many more options. Besides making use of the mineral balancing system, you can go on a low-glycemic-load (GL) diet, which lowers BP remarkably effectively, as the case of David in Chapter 8 illustrates. I have many similar cases of people reporting that their blood pressure has normalised since following a low-GL diet. In addition, this approach is very likely to bring other health benefits, and it's very unlikely to raise your risk of heart attack, unlike diuretics, or cause a nasty persistent dry cough, as can be the case with ACE inhibitors.

The diet favoured by ill-informed doctors and dieticians to lower BP is the 'healthy balanced diet' which usually means a low-fat, high-carbohydrate diet. All too often, though, this allows quite large amounts of sugar, either in fruit juice drinks or in supermarket low-fat meals. A high-sugar diet creates compounds known as aldehydes in the body, which in turn can mess up various proteins that are necessary for calcium channels to work properly; one of the results of this is raised blood pressure.[14]

A version of the low-fat/high-carb diet often used for lowering BP is known as the DASH diet. It recommends the likes of pasta, rice and potatoes, all of which raise blood sugar levels, which in turn raise your insulin levels. Raised insulin levels stimulate the sympathetic nervous system, the one that primes you for action, which in turn releases a chemical that tightens the arteries. Too much insulin also encourages the body to hold on to both salt and water, which also raises blood pressure.[15]

To avoid the BP-raising potential of sugar and other refined carbohydrates the best option is the low-GL diet (see Chapter 8 for the full story), which is why the foundation of my Heart-friendly Diet in Part 4 is low GL. In a small trial the Holford team ran on 16 volunteers on my low-GL diet, blood pressure dropped by 6 points in eight weeks.[16]

For even better results, include various antioxidant-rich nutrients, such as vitamin C and CoQ_{10}, and nutrient-rich foods, plus the key minerals, such as potassium and magnesium, that specifically lower blood pressure, as we saw in Chapters 12 and 13.

Increase magnesium and potassium, and avoid salt

Most of us get about three times as much sodium from salt as we do potassium, when the balance should be about 1:1, so cut back on salt and go for fruit and green leafy vegetables, along with nuts and seeds, which are all rich in both potassium and magnesium.

Just increasing potassium in this way is estimated to drop high blood pressure by 10 per cent.[17] In South Africa, where almost one in four of the black population has hypertension, a recent study found that making simple changes to the diet for eight weeks resulted in a significant reduction in blood pressure.[18] By including six commonly eaten food items in which sodium was decreased and potassium, magnesium and calcium were increased, researchers found it was possible to reduce systolic blood pressure by 6.2mmHg in those with moderate hypertension and already on anti-hypertensive medication, with significant reductions occurring by week four.

There's one kind of salt that's naturally very high in magnesium and potassium, with 61 per cent less sodium; it's called Solo sea salt. It is by far the best-tasting 'healthy' salt. People with high blood pressure given this salt had a decrease in blood pressure, according to a study published in the *British Medical Journal*.[19]

I also recommend you supplement with about 300mg of magnesium. You'll get about 100mg in a good multivitamin, so that means supplementing an additional 200mg.

Also, don't forget to drink plenty of water – six glasses, or about 1 litre (1¾ pints) a day. Drinking water helps, because a lack of it makes the sodium level inside the cells go up, which raises blood pressure.

The benefits of beetroot

One paper recommended beetroot as an effective way of lowering BP.[20] That's because it contains high levels of nitrate, which your saliva turns into nitrites, and these, in turn, are used to make nitric oxide, a gas that dilates the blood vessels and so lowers BP, as we have already seen. Other good sources of nitrate include those dark green leafy vegetables again, celery, lettuce, spinach and radishes. Green leafy vegetables are also a rich source of folate, which lowers homocysteine and cardiovascular risk, again lowering blood pressure. (Chapter 10 gives you the full story on this.)

Remember to have sufficient omega-3

One of the cardiovascular benefits of oily fish is that it is good for lowering blood pressure. If you are getting your omega-3 from a supplement, it's the DHA, and possibly the DPA, rather than the EPA, that relaxes the arteries the most. It does this partly by increasing the levels of nitric oxide and by thinning the blood by stopping the platelets in the blood from clumping together.[21]

Increase your antioxidants

As you may remember, antioxidants help to combat oxidative stress (that is, the cellular damage that occurs due to internal biochemical reactions and external pollutants such as smoke or eating fried food). High levels of oxidative stress are associated with high blood pressure.[22]

Seek out foods rich in bioflavonoids such as berries, cherries, grapes, red wine, green tea and citrus rind, which have been shown to lower BP in animals. Anthocyanidins, which are found in especially high quantities in blue and red fruits, have been shown to relax arteries. I recommend having a daily shot of Cherry Active (Montmorency cherry concentrate).

Also, in one study the dietary supplement pycnogenol, an antioxidant derived from pine bark, was found to allow half a group of 48 diabetics to control their BP and raise nitric oxide levels.[23]

So I'd recommend taking an all-round antioxidant supplement, plus eating antioxidant-rich foods, and seeing what effect that has.

As we saw in Chapter 12, both vitamin C (2g a day) and CoQ_{10} (usually given at a dose of 90mg a day) lower blood pressure. In a joint study by the University of Austin, Texas, and the Centre for Adult Diseases in Osaka, Japan, 52 patients with high blood pressure were treated either with CoQ_{10} or a placebo.[24] There was an 11 per cent decrease in blood pressure for those on CoQ_{10}, compared to a 2 per cent decrease for those on a placebo. In another trial, from 2001, 60mg of CoQ_{10} given twice daily for 12 weeks helped promote normal blood pressure levels by reducing systolic blood pressure.[25] A controlled clinical trial published in 2002, meanwhile, showed that supplementation with 200mg of CoQ_{10} a day helps to promote normal blood pressure levels.[26]

Increase your intake of vitamin D

In addition to the above, aim for a high intake – at least three or four times the RDA – of vitamin D, because hypertension is linked with low levels of vitamin D and raised calcium in cells; one of the roles of vitamin D is to control calcium absorption.[27] You should supplement at least 15mcg a day, especially in the winter.

Check and lower your homocysteine level

High homocysteine is associated with hypertension and I've had many clients with high homocysteine whose blood pressure has rapidly normalised when their homocysteine level comes down. I'm not aware of any studies testing this effect yet but, interestingly, both ACE inhibitors and beta blocker drugs lower homocysteine.[28] I'd certainly recommend you test your homocysteine level (ask your doctor or get a home-test kit – see Resources). If your level is high, supplement a combination of homocysteine-lowering nutrients (see Chapters 10 and 22).

Valda, aged 73, is an interesting example:

Case Study: Valda

Valda had suffered from high blood pressure for over 30 years, as well as a touch of arthritis. Her doctor had given her two drugs, Captopril and a junior aspirin every day. They had helped a bit, but her blood pressure was still high – averaging 150/85.

She decided to have a homocysteine test. Her H score was 43, putting her in the very high-risk category. She started eating more greens and beans, high in folate, and took a homocysteine-lowering supplement.

After two months she was re-tested and her H score had dropped by 88 per cent to a healthy 5.1. Her blood pressure had also dropped and stabilised at 130/80 and she was able to reduce her medication. Her arthritis had also improved with much less joint pain and she felt better in herself.

Master your stress level and exercise every day

Various forms of stress push up your BP by raising the levels of hormones like adrenalin and cortisol, which then constrict the arteries and speed up the heart rate. Meditation and biofeedback both have their supporters as ways to combat stress, and in 2008 there were also positive results reported for 'laughter yoga'. You laugh for 45 seconds and then do deep breathing and stretching, repeat for 20 minutes.[29] In Chapter 24 I'll show you how to reduce your stress load.

Also, don't forget to exercise every day. Something that gets you puffing and panting will help strengthen the heart, relax the arteries and reduce stress. (You'll find more on this in Chapter 23.)

Monitor yourself

Given all the different options for lowering blood pressure, it makes sense to buy yourself a blood pressure monitor to see if what you are doing is having an effect. That's just what the American Heart Association has recommended. Try it and experiment. I'm sure you'll find the right combination of factors to bring your blood pressure under control.

Blood pressure-lowering foods

Eat plenty of the bioflavonoid-rich foods, such as berries, cherries, grapes, red wine (limit to one glass a day), green tea and citrus rind, which have been found to lower BP in animals.

Dark chocolate, or cocoa, also works. Eating about 30 calories a day of dark chocolate was associated with a lowering of blood pressure, without weight gain or other adverse effects, according to a study in the *Journal of the American Medical Association*.[30] That's the equivalent of about two small pieces of a 70 per cent cocoa chocolate, ideally low in sugar or sweetened with xylitol (a natural sweetener that is very low in GLs).

Summary

To lower your blood pressure:

- Eat a low-GL diet, with plenty of fresh fruit and vegetables, including beetroot, pumpkin seeds or chia seeds, and a little bit of chocolate. Eat oily fish for your essential omegas.
- Drink at least 1 litre (1¾ pints) of water a day, a shot of Cherry Active and a small amount of alcohol, especially good-quality wine, and particularly if you are stressed.
- Get your stress levels under control (see Chapter 24).
- Make sure your daily supplement programme includes omega-3, at least 15mcg of vitamin D, 2g of vitamin C and 90mg of CoQ_{10} and a good all-round antioxidant complex.
- Check your homocysteine level and, if raised, lower it with specific high-dose homocysteine-lowering nutrients (see Chapter 10).
- Exercise for at least half an hour a day.

Chapter 22 helps you build your own supplement programme.

CHAPTER 19

Easing Angina and Recovering from a Heart Attack

I f you know you have significant arterial blockages or you have had a heart attack, possibly leaving your heart muscle somewhat compromised, all the prevention steps I've spoken about may be good but not enough for you to make big improvements in your health; however, do not underestimate the combined effect of a total nutritional strategy, ideally personalised by a nutritional therapist (see Resources for details on how to find one) depending on your test results. These steps are also worth taking if you are facing bypass surgery.

A total nutritional strategy may include:

- Following a low-GL diet, with plant sterols, soluble fibres and antioxidant nutrients.

- Taking high-potency niacin for lowering cholesterol and lipoprotein(a) and raising HDL.

- Supplementing with extra antioxidants, including CoQ_{10}, alpha-lipoic acid, vitamin C, vitamin E and glutathione or NAC.

- Extra lysine, especially if your lipoprotein(a) level is raised.

- Extra omega-3s both from eating fish and from supplements.

- Extra magnesium and potassium, and strict sodium avoidance, eating more fruit and veg and supplementing 300mg of magnesium, which relaxes arteries.

The above list forms the basis of the diet and supplementary recommendations in Part 4, together with building up exercise and learning techniques such as HeartMath for reducing your stress level.

Together, these actions have been shown to reduce angina, relax arteries, lower triglycerides and LDLs and reduce the risk of a heart attack; however, there are a few other strategies that you might like to consider.

Boost your nitric oxide level

As you saw in Chapter 2, your body produces a highly versatile nutrient, nitric oxide (NO), that does many of the things you need to recover after a heart attack and improve the health of your arteries. It expands blood vessels, it stops platelets in the blood clumping together forming clots and it helps to break down arterial plaque and, acting as an antioxidant, it helps to protect blood fats from damage.

Although a number of drugs, notably Viagra and ACE inhibitors, aim to boost NO, according to Louis Ignarro (who won a Nobel Prize for his research into NO), you can increase your body's ability to make it by taking a combination of certain supplements as well as exercising. He recommends:

- **L-arginine**, which is an amino acid found in all protein foods. From arginine the body makes NO. He recommends supplementing 2,000–3,000mg taken twice daily (giving a total of 4,000–6,000mg).

- **L-citrulline** Supplemental arginine doesn't enter cells readily unless it is combined with L-citrulline, another amino acid. Melons and cucumbers are rich sources of L-citrulline, but they don't provide high enough levels to significantly increase nitric oxide levels. He recommends 400–600mg daily.

- **A daily multivitamin including vitamin E** Vitamin E helps reduce the assault of cell-damaging free radicals on the endothelial lining and may promote higher levels of nitric oxide. The amount of vitamin E that is in most multivitamin–mineral supplements is about 50iu, which is an effective dose.

- **Vitamin C** Like vitamin E, vitamin C will reduce oxidation in the blood vessels and may cause an increase in nitric oxide. He recommends supplementing at least 500mg.

Some supplements contain all these nutrients as natural NO boosters and they are worth trying if my first-line favourites, outlined above and at the end of this chapter, haven't succeeded in controlling your blood pressure.

Exercise, which also helps boost your own natural levels of NO, needs to be part of your heart-friendly action plan.

CoQ$_{10}$ plus carnitine – the dynamic duo

In Chapter 12 we learnt about the importance of CoQ$_{10}$ for heart-muscle function. If you've had a heart attack, especially if there is some residual damage, CoQ$_{10}$ can really help recovery if taken in combination with the amino acid L-carnitine.

Like CoQ$_{10}$, carnitine is a semi-essential nutrient. This means that your body can make it, but it doesn't make enough for optimal health – especially if you're getting on in years.

Carnitine is made from two amino acids: L-lysine and L-methionine; however, it's better to get a direct supply, especially for heart-muscle function. More than half of your heart's energy comes from fat, and since it's working hard every second, it needs a steady supply. Carnitine is the delivery boy that brings in fatty acids to process for energy. It also takes away the toxic by-products, including damaged fats.

Carnitine helps your heart to liberate the energy it needs efficiently. Without enough, your heart would struggle to function properly, causing heart and blood pressure irregularities. Toxic waste would also accumulate, leading to reduced blood flow (ischaemia), particularly in the legs.

A number of studies confirm its usefulness particularly if there's stress on the heart; for example, after a heart attack or heart failure, or if you suffer from angina. In a study of 47 patients with chronic stable angina given 2g a day of L-carnitine or placebo for three months, those receiving L-carnitine recovered more quickly and showed sufficient improvement to be able to start exercising.[31] In another study, people with coronary artery disease were given both L-carnitine and the antioxidant alpha-lipoic acid for eight weeks, during which time their blood pressure decreased and the diameter of the brachial artery increased, indicating better circulation.[32] Very high doses (9g a day for six days intravenously, followed by 6g a day orally) also help recovery after bypass surgery. A trial on 537 patients showed that propionyl-L-carnitine improves exercise capacity in patients with heart failure and keeps the heart healthy.[33]

The different choices in carnitine

There are actually three different kinds of carnitine, all with slight advantages for different processes in the body. They are:

● L-carnitine

● Acetyl-L-carnitine (ALC)

● Propionyl-L-carnitine (PLC)

All three work in terms of improving heart-muscle function. If you had to pick one, PLC is probably the best. It specifically helps heart- and peripheral-muscle function. It works so well that it's in and out of your heart very quickly, proving the importance of a continuous supply.

L-carnitine and ALC are probably better for brain function. I'd recommend ALC for people with age-related memory decline or Alzheimer's, or to maximise recovery from a stroke. ALC also targets the eyes and ears, and animal studies show that it can actually improve hearing.

So, PLC is probably the best if you've had a heart attack, have angina, or suffer from intermittent claudication (lower leg pain caused by inadequate blood flow to muscles during exercise). You can purchase PLC on its own, or in carnitine complexes that provide all three types.

The best dosages

Ideally, it's better to take carnitine twice or more a day because it only remains in your body for a few hours. The best dosage depends on your level of health. I recommend taking 250–500mg a day for basic health promotion; that is, if you're essentially healthy and want to stay that way and live a long life. If you are over 50, I recommend 500mg a day, divided into two doses.

If you have one of the above health issues, however – heart-muscle problems, angina, heart attack, memory loss or stroke – I suggest that you double or quadruple the dosage. Take 250–500mg of carnitine three to four times a day. Alongside 30mg of CoQ_{10} taken four times a day, it can work wonders. Although these two nutrients work in different ways, they both support your heart and brain by helping to provide a consistent, high level of energy and by reducing the toxic by-products of energy production.

There really aren't any toxicity concerns with carnitine, and certainly not at these levels; however, if you are taking the higher dosages and have an underactive thyroid, keep an eye on your thyroxine levels in case they go down. On the other hand, if you're on anti-convulsive drugs (such as valproic acid), you'll probably need the higher carnitine dosage, as long-term use of these drugs appears to deplete levels.

Chelation therapy

When significant arterial plaque is present in the body, levels of coronary artery calcium go up. In fact, scans designed to detect this build up of calcium in the arteries are sometimes used to diagnose blockages. A high level of coronary artery calcium is very predictive of a worse outcome in those with cardiovascular disease.

If you are already pulling out all the nutritional stops but not making progress, one way to speed up the breakdown of arterial plaque is chelation therapy, as mentioned in Chapter 12. This involves the infusion of the chelating agent, EDTA, which latches onto calcium in arterial plaque and helps to break it down. It's approved by the FDA (Food and Drug Administration in the US) for treating hypercalcaemia (high calcium in the blood).

A chelation infusion usually takes two hours, and will be carried out a number of times, usually over a two- or three-month period. Chelation therapists also give combinations of nutrients in the intravenous infusion, similar to those I recommend in this book. This is especially important because EDTA also chelates (that is, removes) other beneficial minerals such as magnesium, which must be replaced through supplementation. Vitamin C is also a natural, but weaker, chelating agent that does, however, appear to enhance the effectiveness of EDTA.

Chelation therapy has been around since the 1960s but, despite growing evidence of its effectiveness, it is considered controversial by mainstream medicine. This is hardly surprising since it could be seen as an alternative to bypass surgery, which is one of the most lucrative cardiovascular treatments. By the 1990s there had been 19 studies involving over 22,000 patients with vascular disease, of which 87 per cent had improved following chelation therapy.[34] In one study, 58 out of 65 patients cancelled their scheduled coronary bypass surgery, and 24 out of 27 cancelled amputation following significant improvements in circulation.[35] In another, patients who had blockages in their coronary arteries (stenosis) had a 30 per cent reduction after 30 EDTA infusions.[36]

There are also small placebo-controlled studies that have shown no effect, however. These studies have equally been criticised for faulty design. A more recent study of outcomes of those people who had been given at least 20 infusions of EDTA, often monthly, found a much lower incidence of heart attack, repeated coronary bypass surgery or PTCA (percutaneous transluminal coronary angioplasty) and also fewer deaths.[37]

Chelation therapy is certainly something you might want to consider if other options aren't working or desirable. For experienced doctors practising chelation therapy, see Resources. If you have an open-minded cardiologist or doctor, this is an option you might want to discuss with them.

The first step, however, is to apply an aggressive nutrition and lifestyle strategy as explained in Part 4.

Summary

The key factors you need to address to ease angina and atherosclerosis are:

- Following a low-GL diet, with plant sterols, soluble fibres and antioxidant nutrients, as explained in Chapter 21.
- Supplementing high-potency niacin (at least 500mg twice a day) for lowering cholesterol and lipoprotein(a) and raising HDL.
- Extra antioxidants, including CoQ_{10}, alpha-lipoic acid, vitamin C, vitamin E and glutathione or NAC. In Chapter 22 I'll show you how to build your own supplement programme with the correct doses.
- Extra lysine, 1g, three times a day, especially if your lipoprotein(a) level is raised.
- Extra carnitine, 250–500mg, three to four times a day, ideally with CoQ_{10}.
- Extra omega-3s both from eating fish and from supplements providing 2,000mg of EPA a day.
- Extra magnesium and potassium, and strict sodium avoidance, both eating more fruit and veg and supplementing 300mg of magnesium, which relaxes arteries.

If the above doesn't solve your problems, consider adding a formula designed to lower nitric oxide, and investigate EDTA therapy as an option.

CHAPTER 20

How to Maximise Recovery from a Stroke

All the key prevention steps for minimising your risk for heart disease also apply to strokes and for aiding recovery. Specific known risk factors for stroke include age, high blood pressure, high cholesterol, smoking, diabetes, an abnormal heart rhythm (atrial fibrillation) and a previous TIA (transient ischaemic attack) or mini-stroke, so if you have a combination of these your stroke risk is much increased. There are some groups of people who have a higher risk of stroke. People of Afro-Caribbean origin are twice as likely to have a stroke as someone of European origin, and more likely to have a first stroke at a younger age. Similarly, being of South Asian origin also increases your risk. Middle-aged women have a higher stroke risk than middle-aged men, and women in general are more likely to die from stroke.

Although you can't change your age or ethnic background, the good news is that most of the risk factors can be modified by adopting simple changes in dietary and lifestyle habits. Specific dietary changes and regular exercise can help to improve your cholesterol profile, reduce blood pressure and manage diabetes, so where necessary you can take action and target each of these individually. If you also want to stop smoking and break free from addictive habits, then my book *How to Quit Without Feeling S**t* will give you advice on how to do this.

As we saw in Chapter 5, a stroke happens when there is a disturbance in the brain's blood supply which starves cells of oxygen and leads to cell death and a loss of brain function. The effects are similar whether the stroke is ischaemic (when blood flow is blocked) or haemorrhagic (when blood vessels burst). Much of the damage from stroke is believed to result from the activation of various enzymes that affect phospholipids and essential fats, which are key components of brain cell membranes, and through the generation of oxidants, which promote the death of brain cells. When considering ways to minimise this damage and to recover from a stroke it makes sense to not only improve your intake of phospholipids and essential fats but also to provide a means to mop up these damaging oxidants. This is why choline, lecithin, fish oils, B vitamins and antioxidants should form the backbone of any stroke recovery protocol. I'll discuss these and the evidence supporting their use a bit later.

Reduce your risk and assist recovery

There are five steps to reduce your risk further and maximise your recovery:

1. Lower high blood pressure

High blood pressure is one of the top risk factors and is linked with three-quarters of all strokes. Fortunately, there are lots of ways to reduce it without taking drugs, which have their own associated side effects. These are explained in Chapter 18, so make sure you are doing everything necessary in this regard.

2. Improve your cholesterol

Not everyone who has a stroke has a cholesterol problem. Having a high HDL and low LDL reduces your stroke risk. The B vitamin niacin, for example, in doses of 1,000mg, effectively raises HDL and lowers LDL cholesterol. If you do have a cholesterol problem, follow the advice for lowering cholesterol in Chapter 17.

Although we've talked about the need to manage cholesterol levels to reduce your stroke risk, there's one other thing to consider, because cholesterol actually has a role in stroke recovery. Cholesterol helps by transporting the essential fats, which are needed to create nerve pathways and to repair or replace damaged cells. What's more, having cholesterol that is too low can actually result in muscle and nerve degeneration. So bear this in mind, especially if you've been prescribed a cholesterol-lowering drug as part of your stroke rehabilitation programme. These are sometimes given to people who have perfectly normal cholesterol levels and they may do more harm than good.

3. Reverse diabetes

People with type-2 diabetes have almost double the risk of having a stroke within the first five years of diagnosis.[38] The good news is that type-2 diabetes is a reversible condition, the cornerstone of which is a strict low-GL diet. How to eat in this way is explained in Chapter 21; however, if you are diabetic I recommend you read and follow the diabetes reversal programme in my book *Say No to Diabetes*.

4. Go for fish

Stroke can be regarded as an inflammatory disease, and its risk has been strongly associated with both whole fish and fish oil intake. In the Nurses' Health Study Cohort some women had a reduced risk of stroke and a lower incidence of ischaemic strokes – and this was from eating any type of fish. Similar results were shown in those with a high intake of omega-3 oils.[39] Not only do omega-3 fats decrease inflammation and regulate the amount of fatty triglycerides in your blood, but they also decrease blood clotting and stickiness, 'thinning' the blood and improving blood pressure. Oily fish, a great source of the inflammation-reducing, heart-protective, omega-3 oils EPA and DHA, are an ideal food for improving your cardiovascular health and decreasing your stroke risk and I'd recommend that you eat at least three servings of cold-water fish such as herrings, sardines, mackerel, salmon and pilchards each week. They also help the brain and nervous system to repair, which is essential for building more brain cells and connections.

5. Handle homocysteine

As far as strokes are concerned, lowering homocysteine by taking a combination of vitamins B_6, folic acid, B_{12}, TMG and zinc makes a big difference. If taken for three years, folic acid alone can lower stroke risk by almost a third, according to a recent analysis of all trials published in the *Lancet*. I'd certainly recommend you test your homocysteine level and, if your level is high, supplement a combination of homocysteine-lowering nutrients. Read Chapter 10 for more information on homocysteine. These homocysteine-lowering nutrients improve methylation, which helps to re-wire the brain.

Essential supplements to improve recovery

Although the above will help to reduce your risk of a stroke, what can you do if you have already suffered from one and are hoping to support your recovery? Several supplements have been the subject of much research and are certainly worth including to maximise your recovery.

1. Phospholipids

Phospholipids are a type of fat that play a key part in cell membrane structure and are known to have protective effects in the brain – particularly in acute ischaemic stroke. The damaging effects of stroke result from changes in phospholipid structure, which eventually result in cell death. Choline is an essential nutrient (found in eggs and fish but also synthesised in the body) that is used to make phospholipids, and it's possible that having plenty available could minimise cell damage.

As well as being a structural part of brain cell membranes, choline is also used by the body to form the brain chemical acetylcholine, which is involved in many functions, including muscle control and memory. Several studies have investigated a form of choline called cdp-choline (brand name Citicoline) to determine its effectiveness and safety in stroke recovery. This form of choline is converted into phosphatidyl choline, one of several phospholipids.

In a study of patients who suffered an ischaemic stroke and were given Citicoline every day for six weeks, clear improvements were found in their neurological and overall functioning. The best improvements were gained from higher doses, between 2,000 and 5,000mg per day. In some instances there were further health gains when treatment was continued after the six-week period.[40]

In another study presented at the American Stroke Association's 27th International Stroke Conference, in which the brain was assessed by MRI scans taken 12 weeks after a stroke, researchers found that the area of dead tissue within the brain (the infarct) had increased by only 2 per cent in those receiving 2,000mg cdp-choline each day. Infarct size had increased by 34 per cent in those taking a daily dose of 500mg cdp-choline and by a massive 85 per cent in those receiving a placebo drug.

Dosage appears important, as other studies using lower daily amounts of between 500 and 2,000mg cdp-choline found it to be ineffective in stroke recovery.[41]

A decline in mental performance is also very common and is evident in between a half and three-quarters of people six months after a stroke. Choline may protect against such a decline. In a recent six-month trial, published in *Stroke*, Citicoline prevented cognitive decline in individuals recovering from their first-ever ischaemic stroke.[42]

I recommend you take at least 2,000mg of cdp-choline or per-haps hi-pc choline, which is available in health-food stores, each day to minimise cell death and protect against decline in cognitive function, certainly in the first six months. This amount of choline would be present in two to three teaspoons of hi-pc lecithin (pc here stands for phosphatidyl choline), as one teaspoon provides 1,000mg of phosphatidyl choline.

Lecithin capsules also provide phosphatidyl choline, but you need to take a lot. These are normally 1,200mg per capsule, providing about 350mg of choline, so you'd need six a day to achieve therapeutic levels. As well as its role in supporting brain health, lecithin also helps your body to process cholesterol so it is supportive of cardiovascular health too.

2. Antioxidants

The production of oxidants and the process of oxidation are a normal part of the body's day-to-day metabolic functions. In fact, we have a wide variety of antioxidants in our cells and blood that work to neutralise oxidants so that they don't build up and become harmful. Common antioxidants, which can be obtained from your diet, include vitamins A, C and E, and minerals like selenium. In the case of a stroke, it seems that the body is under great oxidative stress and is producing larger amounts of oxidants. After suffering an ischaemic stroke there are significantly lower levels of antioxidants and antioxidant activity in the blood.[43]

If your antioxidant status was quite high before your stroke, you may have already gained some neuro-protection. In a recent study led by Paula Bickford of the University of South Florida College of Medicine, ischaemic strokes were induced in animals that had eaten regular animal food or food supplemented with either blueberries, the algae spirulina or spinach.[44] They found that the antioxidant-rich diets offered greater neuro-protection resulting in more than halving the area of the brain affected by a stroke and providing faster progress in the recovery of movement. 'The clinical implication is that increasing fruit and vegetable consumption may make a difference in the severity of a stroke,' Bickford says.

What is the impact of antioxidants taken after a stroke? Antioxidants may help stroke victims recover faster due to their anti-inflammatory properties and their ability to quench oxidants, which will still cause brain-cell death three to six days after the initial event; however, although several trials suggest their benefits in stroke recovery, data in human trials is still limited.

Alpha-lipoic acid (ALA) is an antioxidant compound that may reduce inflammation inside the blood vessels, making it possible for your blood vessels to heal after you suffer a stroke. ALA may also help to prevent another stroke. Researchers at the University of Maryland Medical Centre found that animals receiving ALA were four times more likely to survive a stroke and less likely to suffer with brain damage than those that didn't.

Vitamin C may help your blood vessels to heal after a stroke, and it has also been shown to protect against cognitive changes, particularly in those experiencing new cardiovascular events.[45] Furthermore, vitamin C may help protect you from suffering another stroke, since research studies have shown that people with high levels of vitamin C in their bloodstreams have a significantly lower risk of suffering from a stroke than people with low blood levels.[46]

Vitamin E may improve your memory after a stroke and reduce your risk of a second stroke. A study at the Columbia Presbyterian Medical Centre showed that people who took vitamin E supplements reduced their risk of suffering strokes by 53 per cent compared to people who didn't take vitamin E supplements. The study group included many adults who had already suffered at least one stroke.

A meta-analysis in the *British Medical Journal*, however, suggests that vitamin E reduces the common kind of ischaemic stroke but increases risk of the rarer haemorrhagic stroke.[47] I contacted Dr Maret Traber, the vitamin E expert at the Linus Pauling Institute, who knows more about vitamin E than anyone, for her comment on this study and this is what she said:

'The authors highlight both the strengths and limitations of their analysis. Strengths include a large sample size from high quality randomised controlled studies (RCTs) and inclusion of studies that are combinable (i.e. similar design). Some of the limitations include [the fact that] most of the data were derived from studies involving diseased or high risk patients, so the results may not be relevant to the general population. The authors focused solely on stroke outcomes, not addressing other cardiovascular outcomes and other health outcomes. Several individual vitamin E RCTs have shown benefits from supplemental vitamin E on other cardiovascular outcomes beyond stroke, including the Women's Health Study (WHS) and the Women's Antioxidant Cardiovascular Study (WACS). Supplemental vitamin E may also provide benefits beyond cardiovascular events, including immune function and eye health. This meta-analysis did not address these other important and relevant outcomes.

'This analysis only examined RCTs involving supplemental vitamin E alone. We know that antioxidants (and indeed all nutrients) don't function in isolation but as part of complex networks, so the idea that a single nutrient, supplemented at high doses in primarily cardiovascular patients or smokers, will have potent effects may be misplaced to begin with. Even though many studies (including those examined in this analysis) show benefits of supplemental vitamin E, it may be wiser to examine vitamin E's effects in the context of the full antioxidant network, rather than in isolation.

'The authors also acknowledge that, although the relative risk numbers appear high (22% increase for hemorrhagic and 10% decrease for ischemic, respectively), the absolute effects are quite small and may be somewhat misleading, placing in question the clinical relevance of this report. Based on their analysis, the authors estimate that for every 1000 patients exposed to vitamin E they would predict 0.8 more hemorrhagic strokes and 2.1 fewer ischemic strokes. So the benefits may actually outweigh the risks, when it comes to stroke.'

There are two other points worth bearing in mind. We know that statin drugs, widely prescribed to those with cardiovascular risk, knock out CoQ_{10}, which is needed for vitamin E to function as an antioxidant. There is no way of knowing what percentage of people in these trials where taking both statins and high-dose vitamin E, which I never recommend *unless* you are also supplementing 90mg of CoQ_{10}.

Also, vitamin E has anti-atherosclerotic and antiplatelet effects that may reduce the rate of ischaemic stroke. On the other hand, vitamin E exerts an anticoagulant effect via inhibition of vitamin K-dependent clotting-factors activation. If a person were on both blood-thinning drugs, especially warfarin, and high-dose vitamin E, maybe this is too much thinning. It is wise to limit vitamin E if you are on these drugs. See page 65 for more on this subject.

Also, most people are not achieving even basic levels of vitamin E. In reality, supplementing 100 or 200mg of vitamin E is likely to confer protection. That's what I take daily.

In summary, I recommend taking an all-round antioxidant supplement twice a day that provides a combination of antioxidants, ideally including alpha-lipoic acid, glutathione or NAC, vitamin E, the potent plant antioxidant resveratrol and CoQ_{10}. Take with at least 2g of vitamin C for additional support.

3. Fish and fish oils

Fish contains the omega-3 oils EPA and DHA which are integral for brain development and repair, and by lowering triglycerides, blood pressure and arrhythmias they are also vital for a healthy heart. EPA and DHA also help to reduce depression, which is very common after a stroke. Almost one in two stroke survivors will experience post-stroke depression (PSD) at some stage in the first few years, perhaps experiencing symptoms such as social withdrawal and loss of pleasure in previously enjoyed hobbies and activities or life in general, irritability and restlessness, frequent crying episodes, sleep disturbances, fatigue and lethargy, self-loathing or an overwhelming sense of hopelessness. PSD is considered as the most common and important emotional outcome of stroke but it is often overlooked.[48] According to Eoin Redahan, a director of the Stroke Association,

'Wider recognition of depression would lead to an increase in those being treated which is vital ... Evidence shows that those with depression appear to recover less well after a stroke compared to those who do not have depression.'

For these reasons I recommend you eat omega-3-rich oily fish (salmon, mackerel, herring, sardines or trout), two to three times a week. Vegetable sources of omega-3s include raw, unsalted seeds and nuts. The best seeds are chia and flax. You will get more goodness out of them by grinding them first and sprinkling them on cereal, soups and salads. Also use cold-pressed seed oils on salads and vegetables. Choose an oil blend containing flaxseed oil for salad dressings and cold uses, such as drizzling on vegetables instead of butter. Don't cook with these oils as their fats are easily damaged by heat. Walnuts are also rich in omega-3.

I also recommend supplementing omega-3 fish oils; however, because these also help to thin the blood, caution is required if you are on blood-thinning drugs. See page 65 for more on this subject.

4. B vitamins for methylation

Methylation, a vital process for nerve repair, is indicated by your homocysteine level, so this should be a standard test for anyone who has had a stroke. While supplements of just folic acid also lower stroke risk,[49] I don't recommend you take a single folic acid supplement because it can mask a B_{12} deficiency – and insufficient B_{12} is very common, especially later in life.

I'd therefore advise you to supplement folic acid, B_{12} and B_6, together with TMG and zinc, as well as N-acetyl cysteine (this further improves methylation) and to continue doing so in the long term if you have suffered a stroke. (Homocysteine levels tend to revert to their original values after ten weeks without supplementation.)[50] The best formulas contain all of these. But first, test your homocysteine level. Stroke risk increases from a level of 10mcmol/l. The supplemental levels you need, depending on your homocysteine level, are explained in Chapter 22.

Stroke recovery takes time

Stroke affects everyone differently and the level of recovery cannot be predicted. Much recovery occurs in the first few weeks while a person is still in hospital, but improvements may also occur over a number of years. But what does it mean to recover from a stroke? For many it is a combination of acquiring new skills and relearning old ones, learning to adapt to limitations and receiving social, emotional and practical support. This could be achieved by exploring comprehensive-holistic treatment, considering active, problem-based coping strategies, and receiving support from families and health-care professionals.

The brain is a sensitive and complicated organ, and recovering from a stroke will take time. If you can, tailor your recovery programme to best suit your individual needs, and please don't waste a single moment worrying about the speed of your rehabilitation. Just make sure that you are achieving optimum brain nutrition and let nature take its course.

If a person is having difficulty swallowing, making taking supplements a challenge, an alternative would be a nutrient-rich shake such as Get Up & Go (see Resources), with added hi-pc lecithin and ground chia seeds, plus piercing a capsule of omega-3 fish oils. Vitamin capsules or tablets can be crushed and added to food.

Summary

To maximise recovery:

- If you have high blood pressure, you need to bring this down. Certainly include daily supplementation of 300mg of magnesium. Also read Chapter 18.
- If you have high cholesterol and low HDL cholesterol, also supplement 1,000mg of slow-release or non-blushing niacin. Read Chapter 17.

- Increase your intake of oily fish to three times a week and also take two fish oil capsules a day providing 1,000mg of EPA. If you are on blood-thinning medication you need to discuss this with your doctor, because you may need less medication since omega-3 fats are also good for reducing blood thickness.
- Check your homocysteine level. If it is high, you need to supplement high-dose B vitamins in a specific homocysteine-lowering formula. This is explained in Chapter 22. Also read Chapter 10 for other diet and lifestyle tips for lowering homocysteine.
- To aid brain recovery have 3 teaspoons of a high phosphatidyl choline lecithin or the equivalent of 500mg of cdp-choline a day. You can sprinkle this over your breakfast. Alternatively, take six lecithin capsules a day.
- Increase your intake of antioxidants in two ways: firstly, by eating a lot more fresh vegetables, fruits, herbs and spices, choosing a range of brightly coloured foods. See Chapter 12 for more details on this. Chapter 21 includes these foods in your Heart-friendly Diet. Secondly, add an antioxidant complex to your daily supplement programme. Choose one that includes alpha-lipoic acid, glutathione or NAC, vitamin E, the potent plant antioxidant resveratrol and CoQ_{10}. Take with at least 2g of vitamin C for additional support.

Chapter 22 helps you build your own supplement programme.

PART 4

YOUR HEART-FRIENDLY ACTION PLAN

Whether you have heart disease or you want to make sure that you never get it, this part explains what to do to keep your cardiovascular system in top condition. You'll learn the key diet factors and how to apply these with straightforward daily menus and recipes. You will be able to create your own perfect supplement programme either for prevention or to reverse your current health issues. You'll also be able to create a practical and doable strategy for exercise and stress reduction, which are other key pieces of your Heart-friendly Action Plan.

CHAPTER 21

Your Heart-friendly Diet

The key to preventing and reversing heart disease is to provide all the right nutrients your cardiovascular system relies on to stay healthy and to avoid those that cause problems. By emphasising those foods that are good for you there's not so much room for the less desirable foods. The basic principles that I've taken into account in devising your Heart-friendly Diet are as follows:

1. Eat the right diet

The most effective nutritional approach means eating a low-GL diet that includes plenty of oats, barley and beans, and vegetables like okra, aubergines, kale and spinach to get plenty of soluble fibre, folic acid and magnesium. Also use turmeric, garlic and ginger liberally in your cooking. Avoid sugar, deep-fried foods and salt (except for Solo sea salt, which is high in magnesium). Cut back on meat, cheese and other high-fat foods, especially if they are fried.

2. Include plenty of healthy fats

For omega-3 fats, think fish. Have three servings a week of oily fish such as mackerel, wild or organic salmon, herrings or sardines. If you are vegetarian then seeds and nuts will be your main source of omega-3 fats. Chia, flax or pumpkin seeds are all good choices. They can be ground or eaten whole. Try my four-seed mix, which can be sprinkled over breakfast, salads or stir-fries or mixed into yoghurt as a snack. Alternatively, just have a dessertspoonful of chia seeds a day whether or not you are vegetarian.

Four-seed mix

1   Fill a glass jar that has a sealing lid half with chia or flax seeds (rich in omega-3) and half with sesame and sunflower (rich in omega-6) and pumpkin seeds (rich in omega-6 plus omega-3).
2   Keep the jar sealed and in the fridge to minimise damage from light, heat and oxygen.
3   Put a handful in a coffee or seed grinder; grind up and put a tablespoon onto your cereal. Store the remainder in the fridge and use over the next few days.

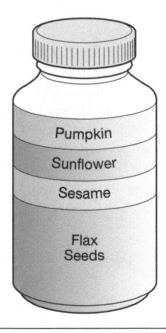

3. Get to know the plant sterols

Soya (as tofu or soya milk, for example), as well as almonds, seeds, oats, lentils and beans will provide you with plenty of the cholesterol-busting plant sterols. Eat sterol-rich foods every day. A small serving of tofu, about 50g (1¾oz) of soya, will give you 2.5g of plant sterols, your daily goal. The best foods for plant sterols are listed in the table below. So you could, for example, eat a soya burger for lunch or serve a salmon, broccoli and sesame seed steam-fry (see page 231) alongside a portion of brown rice and easily reach your daily target of plant sterols. Although cooking doesn't significantly decrease the amount of sterols in a food, try to include a mix of both raw and cooked sterol-rich foods.

Best foods for plant sterols

	Food source	Total plant sterol content (mg/100g fresh weight)
Whole grains	Oat flakes	45
	Wheat germ	345
	Wheat bran	200
	Brown rice	87
Legumes	Peas	135
	Beans	127
Nuts and seeds	Peanuts	117
	Almonds	138
	Walnuts	108
	Pecan nuts	108
	Pistachio nuts	108
Vegetables	Beetroot	25
	Broccoli	37
	Cauliflower	31
	Brussels sprouts	37
	Leek	19
	Dill	32
	Parsley	28
	Peas	30
	Red pepper	22
	Sweetcorn (frozen)	28
	Alfalfa shoots	20

	Alfalfa seeds	196
Fruits	Apples	18
	Avocados	75
	Blueberries	26
	Raspberries	27
	Green grapes	20
	Kiwi	18
	Orange	23
Oils	Rice bran	1055
	Corn	952
	Wheat germ	553
	Flax seed	338
	Soybean	221
	Olive	176
	Coconut	91

(Source: V. Piironen, et al., 'Plant sterols in vegetables, fruit and berries', *Journal of the Science of Food and Agriculture*, 2003; 83(4): 330–337)

4. Eat greens and beans to lower homocysteine

As well as eating plenty of greens, nuts, seeds and beans, which are rich in folic acid and vitamin B_6, include some fish, lean meat, eggs or milk as sources of vitamin B_{12} – all rich sources of B vitamins, which are vital for supporting methylation processes and reducing your homocysteine. In any event, make sure you are supplementing a high-strength multivitamin or B complex if you are over 50 or your cholesterol level or LDL level is high, or your HDL level is low. I'll discuss this in detail in Chapter 22, but try to check your homocysteine level first (either ask your doctor for this test or go for a home test kit, see Resources).

5. Ensure your diet is antioxidant rich

Eat lots of fruit and vegetables, fish and seeds to ensure you have a broad supply of antioxidants. As you saw in the table on pages

132–3, Chapter 12, the best antioxidant-rich foods have the strongest colours, so aim to include something orange, yellow, blue/red and dark green every day, ideally achieving 6,000 ORACs, which is any three of the servings shown in the table on pages 132–3.

6. Look at your addictions

If you're quite addicted to coffee, tea, chocolate, alcohol and/or cigarettes, you'll definitely get a better result by stopping these or, at least, cutting back on them. Try halving your daily intake of these stimulants; you might replace coffee and tea with naturally caffeine-free herbal teas or eat a piece of fruit instead of your chocolate bar, for example. If you do eat chocolate, make sure it is dark, 70 per cent cocoa and low in sugar.

Now it's time to get started on your new low-GL diet. Getting ready to start is a bit like a warm-up before you exercise, because you need a week to prepare: to restock your fridge with low-GL foods; find the best alternative foods and drinks and your nearest suppliers; and get used to eating some of the new foods.

Your Heart-friendly Diet

Whether you need to lose weight or you want to care for your heart by eating a healthy diet, the low-GL diet is the same, it's just that if you don't need to lose weight you can have a little more carbohydrate each day. Here is a summary of the main goals, which I recommend you try to meet when planning your own meals:

- **Have three meals a day and two snacks** Aim for 10GLs per main meal and 5GLs per snack. If you do not need to lose weight, you can relax this to 15GLs per main meal and 7.5GLs per snack. You also have an additional 5GLs per day for drinks, making a total of 45GLs for weight loss and 65GLs for general cardiovascular health.

- **Always combine protein and carbohydrate foods** in a meal, to help slow the energy release for better blood sugar balance.

- **Eat multi-coloured foods regularly**, ideally choosing something yellow, orange, blue/red, and green every day.

- **Plan your meals** to ensure that you are eating your 6,000 ORAC recommended daily intake (see pages 132–3).

- **Aim to have at least three servings of oily fish** (such as salmon, mackerel, herring, kippers, tuna) a week, preferably unfried, and four or more servings of fish in total (including white fish) a week.

- **Eat some omega-3-rich raw seeds or nuts** every day, such as a tablespoon of chia or flax seeds, or a small handful of walnuts or pumpkin seeds. You could have a small handful of raw nuts or seeds, perhaps ground and added to your cereal or to soups or as a snack with some fruit. If you are a strict vegetarian or vegan you'll need double this amount.

- **Eat a maximum of six free-range or organic eggs** a week, preferably from chickens fed on omega-3-rich feed.

- **Plan your meals** to ensure you are eating your recommended daily intake of omega-3 fats (explained on page 77).

- **Eat foods rich in methylation-supporting B vitamins** This means eating more wholefoods: nuts, seeds, beans, whole grains and vegetables.

- **Aim for seven servings of fruit and vegetables** a day; for example, fruit with breakfast and two fruit snacks, plus two servings of vegetables with each main meal.

- **Eat plenty of green vegetables**.

- **Eat a serving of soya, beans or lentils** most days. This could be via using beans and pulses in a main meal, using soya milk on your breakfast or simply having a snack of hummus and crudités or oatcakes.

Plan your meals

On the low-GL diet it is important to 'graze rather than gorge'. GLs are distributed during the day to spread out the carbohydrate load and avoid blood sugar dips and peaks. (You will find a list of foods with their GL values in the Appendix of this book.) You have a 5GL quota per day for drinks or desserts – so you will be able to have a low-GL dessert, diluted fruit juice or a small glass of dry wine or spirit if you want to.

What to eat for breakfast

First of all, never skip breakfast. It's the most important meal of your day. When you wake up your blood sugar is low because you haven't eaten, so you need to eat. But many people who are trying to lose weight or to control their weight make the fatal mistake of trying not to eat anything for as long as possible. This is not good news for your heart health. What often happens is that you get through the morning on liquid stimulants (coffee or tea), nicotine, or instant sugar in the form of a piece of toast or a croissant, but as your blood sugar level dips lower and lower you finally buckle under the strain and end up bingeing on high-GL foods.

Avoiding that kind of scenario is why you must eat breakfast. This was tested by nutritionists at Oxford Brookes University who found that children who ate a high-GL breakfast were more hungry at lunchtime and ate more food than those who ate a low-GL breakfast.[1] Exactly the same thing has been shown in adults, too.[2]

The message is clear. Eat a low-GL breakfast. It will satisfy you for longer by keeping your blood sugar level more stable, so you'll eat less later.

There are two ways to do this.

1   The simplest is to choose from any of the low-GL breakfasts listed on pages 214–15. These are already calculated to give you no more than 10GLs, plus the right amount of protein and essential fats.

Breakfast

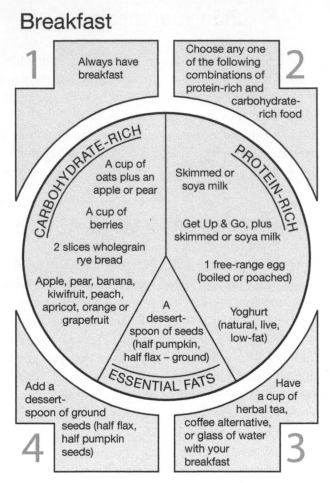

The low-GL breakfast

There are five fundamental breakfasts that give you the correct balance of both carbohydrate and protein. These are:

A balanced breakfast

Carbohydrates		Protein
Cereal/fruit	+	seeds/yoghurt/milk
Fruit	+	yoghurt/seeds
Fruit	+	Get Up & Go/milk

| Bread/toast | + | egg |
| Bread/toast | + | fish (such as kippers) |

We now need to look at the amount you can have of cereal, fruit, toast, and so on. Let's kick off with the cereal-based breakfast, sweetened with fruit rather than sugar.

The best cereal-based breakfasts

A good cereal-based breakfast needs to include a low-GL cereal, a low-GL fruit as a sweetener and a source of protein and essential fats. The goal, remember, is no more than 10GLs. In the chart below you'll see how much of the following six cereals you can have to total 5GLs. As you can see, the best 'value' in terms of your appetite are oat flakes, either cooked as in porridge or eaten raw, just as you would cornflakes. Basically, you could eat as much as you like, given that two servings will fill anybody up.

The GLs for cereal servings

Cereal*	5GLs
Oat flakes	2 servings or cups
All-Bran	1 serving (½ bowl or 1 cup)
Unsweetened muesli	1 small serving (less than ½ bowl or ¾ cup)
Alpen	½ serving (¼ bowl or ½ cup)
Raisin Bran	½ serving (¼ bowl or ½ cup)
Weetabix	1 biscuit

* Adding a dessertspoonful (two teaspoons) of oat bran to your cereal will lower the GL further.

In the following chart you can see how much of these six fruits you could eat to equal 5GLs.

The GLs for fruit servings (breakfast)

Fruit	5GLs
Berries	1 large punnet
Pear	1
Grapefruit	1
Apple	1 small (can fit into the palm of your hand)
Peach	1 small
Banana	less than half

So, your best bet out of the above foods would be to have porridge or raw oat flakes with as many berries as you could eat. Alternatively, you could have a bowl of All-Bran and a grapefruit, or a bowl of unsweetened muesli with a small grated apple. You can also build your own breakfast using the GL chart in the Appendix.

The protein element

As far as protein is concerned, there's some in milk (or in soya milk, but pick the unsweetened kind). Rice milk is high GL and best avoided. Oat milk is not bad, but not as good as soya. Yoghurt (unsweetened) is also high in protein. So, have a spoonful of yoghurt, some milk or some soya milk on your cereal if you'd like to.

Another source of protein, as well as containing countless vitamins, minerals, essential fats and fibre, is seeds. I recommend you have a tablespoon of ground seeds on your cereal as well. Ground chia seeds are the best choice because they are high in both protein and soluble fibres. Flax seeds are the next best thing but not so tasty. Pumpkin seeds are also good, and high in magnesium.

The best yoghurt-based breakfasts

If you are fond of yoghurt, you could dispense with the cereal altogether and have yoghurt, fruit and seeds. In the chart below you'll see how much yoghurt you can eat for 5GLs. (A small pot of yoghurt is 150g/5½oz.)

The GLs for yoghurt servings

Yoghurt	5GLs
Plain yoghurt	2 small pots, 330mg (11½oz)
Non-fat yoghurt	2 small pots, 330mg (11½oz)
Low-fat yoghurt with fruit and sugar	Less than 1 small pot, 100g (3½oz)

So, provided you choose a yoghurt that doesn't have added sugar, you can eat two small pots and sweeten it with any of the fruits you like from the fruit chart above, plus a tablespoon of ground seeds. There is no need to go for the low-fat option.

Breakfasts based on Get Up & Go

Get Up & Go is a powder that you blend with a piece of fruit, choosing from any of the 5GL servings of fruit shown above, and 300ml (10fl oz/ ½ pint) of skimmed milk (or sugar-free soya milk if you prefer).

Get Up & Go is made from a special blend of quinoa, brown rice and soya flour, giving an excellent quality of protein. It is balanced with carbohydrate, mainly from whole apple powder, together with oat bran, rice bran and psyllium husks for added soluble fibre, plus sesame, sunflower and pumpkin seeds and some almond meal, cinnamon and natural vanilla for flavour. In addition, it has added vitamins and minerals, including 50mcg of chromium and 1,000mg of vitamin C, plus all the B vitamins.

When it's made up, Get Up & Go is guaranteed to fill you up until lunchtime, and yet it is only 283 calories and 5GLs. The best fruits to use in Get Up & Go are strawberries, raspberries, a soft pear or blackcurrants (which you can also buy canned in apple juice). You'll be looking for no more than another 5GLs from the fruit you blend in with it. Also add a teaspoon of cinnamon. With dairy or unsweetened soya milk this totals 8GLs. With oat milk it totals 10GLs.

Get Up & Go is available in health-food stores or by mail order (see Resources).

The best egg-based breakfasts

Although it is true that more than half the calories in an egg come from fat, the kind of fat depends on what you feed the chicken. Most eggs come from battery chickens. If you know how unhealthy they are, you won't be keen to eat their eggs, which are high in saturated fat.

On the other hand, there are egg producers in the UK (and many more abroad) that give their chickens feed rich in fatty acids, for example flax seeds. Omega-3-rich free-range or organic eggs are much better for you than ordinary eggs. I recommend you have no more than six free-range or organic eggs a week on my diet – and only these kinds of egg. Have either two small eggs or one large egg at one meal. Poach, boil or scramble them, but don't fry them, since the high heat damages the essential fats.

As eggs are pure protein and fat (so they have a 0GL score), what carbohydrate can you have with them? If this is your entire breakfast you can use up your complete 10GL quota by having any of the following bread servings.

The GLs for bread and bread-substitute servings for breakfast

Bread	10 GLs
Oatcakes	4
Rye 'pumpernickel' style	2 thin slices
Sourdough rye bread	2 thin slices
Rye wholemeal bread (yeasted)	1 slice
Wheat wholemeal bread (yeasted)	1 slice
White, high-fibre bread (yeasted)	less than 1 slice (best avoided)

As you can see, your best 'value' breads are oatcakes, or Scandinavian-style pumpernickel, sonnenbrot- or volkenbrot-type breads, or sourdough rye bread, made without yeast. Sourdough breads, and others like them, are real breads: substantial, fibre-rich and delicious, unlike the light, white, fluffy 'fake' breads mostly on offer, which are full of air, super-refined and nutritionally inferior. You may find the change a bit of a shock at first, but you'll discover that they are very satisfying.

Real breads are better because they have far fewer additives, they use coarsely ground flours and, in the case of sourdough, they have no added yeast. All this keeps the GL score lower.

Some grains are better for you than others because of the type of carbohydrate they contain. The best are oats, followed by barley and rye. Whereas the GL of wheat varies depending on how long you cook it, oats are the same in any shape or form. Whole oat flakes, rolled oats or oatmeal, as used in oatcakes, all have a low glycemic effect.[3]

Kippers, anyone?

Although they have gone out of fashion, kippers (smoked herring) make a fabulous low-GL breakfast, which is tasty and highly nutritious.

Rich in protein and omega-3 fats, one kipper and any of the bread portions shown above will meet your needs for a healthy breakfast.

What to eat for lunch and dinner

Main meals are really something to look forward to on my low-GL diet, but how do you put it all together? The easiest way to get the right nutritional balance is to imagine all the different foods on a plate using the method described below.

Half the plate will consist of very low-GL vegetables. This includes peas, broccoli, runner beans, courgettes and kale, among many others. These vegetables, listed on page 223, will account for no more than 4GLs, and I'm going to show you how to cook them in minutes. If you haven't been all that interested in veg up to now, you'll be amazed by how fresh and zingy they can taste when they're cooked in these ways.

The other half of your plate is divided into two, one for protein-based food such as meat, fish or tofu, and the other for more 'starchy' vegetables, which account for 6–7GLs. So, a quarter of what's on your plate is protein-rich, a quarter is carbohydrate-rich and half is made up of very low-GL vegetables. You'll soon get the hang of it; it's very simple.

More fish, less meat

Let's kick off with the protein serving on your plate. The overall amount of protein – by which I mean the protein contained in the various foods – needs to be at least 20g (¾oz) for each meal. The protein-rich food on your plate will provide 15g (½oz) of this, and the table below tells you how much you need to eat of each of these to get that 15g (½oz). (The one serving of carbohydrate-rich starchy vegetables and two servings of very low-GL vegetables will provide the remaining 5g/⅛oz.)

In the table I've listed a lot of fish options and fewer meat options. In fact, red meat is missing entirely. White meat tends to be much lower in fat, and fish is much higher in the essential omega-3 fats, so becoming a 'fishichicketarian' is a great way to improve cardiovascular health and even lose weight. Does this mean you can never eat red meat? Certainly not, but do stick to lean meat.

How big is a protein serving?

Food	Weight	Serving
Tofu and tempeh	160g (5¾oz)	¾ packet
Soya mince	100g (3½oz)	3 tbsp
Chicken (no skin)	50g (1¾oz)	1 very small breast
Turkey (no skin)	50g (1¾oz)	½ small breast
Quorn	120g (4¼oz)	⅓ pack
Salmon and trout	55g (2oz)	1 very small fillet
Tuna (canned in brine)	50g (1¾oz)	¼ can
Sardines (canned in brine)	75g (2¾oz)	⅔ can
Cod	65g (2¼oz)	1 very small fillet
Clams	60g (2⅛oz)	¼ can
Prawns	85g (3oz)	6 large prawns
Mackerel	85g (3oz)	1 medium fillet
Oysters	–	15
Yoghurt (natural, low fat)	285g (10oz)	½ large tub
Cottage cheese	120g (4¼oz)	½ medium tub
Hummus	200g (7oz)	1 small tub
Skimmed milk	440ml	about 15fl oz (¾ pint)
Soya milk	415ml	about 15fl oz (¾ pint)
Eggs (boiled)	–	2
Quinoa	125g (4½oz)	large serving bowl
Baked beans	310g (11oz)	¾ can
Kidney beans	175g (6oz)	⅓ can
Black-eye beans	175g (6oz)	⅓ can
Lentils	165g (5¾oz)	⅓ can

Starchy vegetables

As we've seen on the plate above, carbohydrate-rich starchy vegetable servings should be roughly the same size or weight as protein servings, but this does depend on how each food weighs up; for example, if you are eating chicken with rice, the serving size of rice is some-what larger than the piece of chicken for each to be roughly the same weight because chicken is dense and heavy and rice is relatively light.

Remember, starchy vegetables will account for a maximum of 7GLs of your meal (out of a total of 10GLs). Let's take a look at what quantity of different starchy vegetables you can eat to keep within that limit, leaving 3GLs for the very low-GL veg that occupy half the plate.

The GLs for starchy vegetables

Starchy vegetables	7GLs
Pumpkin/squash	big serving, 185g (6¾oz)
Carrot	1 large, 160g (5¾oz)
Swede	big serving, 150g (5½oz)
Quinoa	big serving, 130g (4½oz)
Beetroot	big serving, 110g (3¾oz)
Cornmeal	serving, 115g (4oz)
Pearl barley	small serving, 95g (3¼oz)
Wholemeal pasta	½ serving, 85g (3oz) cooked weight
White pasta	⅓ serving, 65g (2¼oz) cooked weight
Brown rice	small serving, 70g (2½oz) cooked weight
White rice	⅓ serving, 45g (1½oz) cooked weight
Couscous	⅓ serving, 45g (1½oz) soaked weight
Broad beans	serving, 30g (1oz)
Corn on the cob	½ cob, 60g (2⅛oz)
Boiled potato	3 small potatoes, 75g (2¾oz)
Baked potato	½ potato, 60g (2⅛oz)
French fries	tiny portion, 45g (1½oz)
Sweet potato	½ potato, 60g (2⅛oz)

As you can see, there are some obvious winners. Wholemeal pasta and brown rice are much better than white pasta and white rice. (Brown basmati rice has the lowest GL score of all the different types of rice.) Swede, carrot and squash are much better than potato. Boiled potato is better than baked potato, which is better than French fries.

Some of these foods may be new to you. If so, try the nutty flavour of quinoa and the smooth, rich savour of the squashes. If you love pasta, switching to the wholemeal variety is painless. They cook the same, but you can eat more of the unrefined variety and stay slim and healthy.

Beans and lentils

It's telling that beans and lentils are no longer widely eaten in many of the world's fattest nations. These are the best foods for both balancing your blood sugar and giving the right mix of protein and carbohydrate. It's this rare double-whammy that keeps their GL score low. (Another reason why lentils and soya – a bean that is more usually eaten as tofu or milk – are so low in GIs is that they contain a substance that prevents the digestion of amylose, therefore slowing down its release further.) As we know, soya keeps your arteries healthy by lowering the 'bad' LDL cholesterol. A serving of soya a day, either as soya milk or tofu, can lower your LDL cholesterol by over 10 per cent.

If your meal contains beans and lentils you can be quite generous with the portion size because you are getting both the protein and the carbohydrate from the same food; however, when you are eating these foods as your source of protein, combine with only half the serving size of a carbohydrate-rich food, instead of an equal serving. If you were making a lentil casserole for two people, for example, you'd use a cup of uncooked lentils and half a cup of uncooked brown rice. This is, of course, because you're already getting a significant amount of carbohydrate in the lentils.

The chart below shows how much you can eat, assuming you are not eating another starchy vegetable, to stay within 7GLs. (Most regular cans of beans provide around 225–245g (8–8½oz).)

The GLs for beans, chickpeas and lentils

Beans and lentils	7 GLs
Soya beans	2 cans
Pinto/borlotti beans	¾ can
Lentils	¾ can
Baked beans	½ can
Butter beans	½ can
Split peas	½ can
Kidney beans	½ can
Chickpeas	⅓ can

NOTE A 400g (14oz) can is roughly equivalent to 75g (3oz) dried beans.

If you're not vegetarian, you may be relatively unfamiliar with beans and lentils. You may have encountered dhal, baked beans, hummus or cassoulet, but never actually thrown a packet or tin of lentils or beans into your shopping basket. These are great foods, immensely satisfying in flavour and texture, and they feature in all of the world's great cuisines – as well as kitchen classics such as beans on toast.

Eat your food slowly

Chew each mouthful 20 times, as this will further 'slow-release' the carbohydrate in your food. Also, sip water with your meal.

Non-starchy vegetables

Now it's time to move on to the other half of your plate. This is made up of what I call the 'unlimited vegetables', although there are, of course, some limits, but these are vegetables for which a serving is less than 2 GLs. A serving of peas, for instance, is a cupful.

Non-starchy vegetables

Asparagus	Cucumber	Onions
Aubergine	Endive	Peas
Beansprouts	Fennel	Peppers
Broccoli	Garlic	Radish
Brussels sprouts	Green beans and runner beans	Rocket
Cabbage	Kale	Spinach
Cauliflower	Lettuce	Spring onions
Celery	Mangetouts	Tomato
Courgette	Mushrooms	Watercress

If you are not a fan of cabbage, say, or runner beans I hope you will change your mind when you read some of my cooking recommendations, such as steam-frying, which adds lots of flavour and keeps vegetables crisp and fresh. They are brimming with vitamins, minerals and other phytonutrients so they are really good for you. Aim to eat at least half your vegetables raw or lightly cooked or steamed. Cooking, burning or frying generates more oxidants (see page 230).

To recap, I want you to eat two servings of non-starchy vegetables, one serving of starchy vegetables and one serving of protein-based food. Together, they'll help you feel full at the end of every meal.

What to eat for snacks

Research shows clearly that 'grazing' (eating little and often) is healthier for you than 'gorging' (having one or two big meals in the day).[4] Grazing helps keep your blood sugar level even, and this makes overeating far less likely, as you'll never experience any between-meal hunger pangs. For this reason I recommend you have a mid-morning and a mid-afternoon snack, because it helps to keep your blood sugar level stable. The ideal snack is one that provides no more than 5GLs and also some protein, and the simplest snack food is fruit, eaten with nuts or seeds. Let's see what you'd need to eat to stay within 5GLs for your snack.

The GLs for fruit servings (snacks)

Fruit	5GLs
Strawberries	1 large punnet
Plums	4
Cherries	1 small punnet
Pear	1
Grapefruit	1
Orange	1
Apple	1 small (can fit into the palm of your hand)
Peach	1 small
Melon/watermelon	1 slice

Berries, plums and cherries are your best 'value' fruit snacks. Berries include raspberries, blueberries, blackberries and any others that you can get your hands on in season. You can further lower the GL score of these fruits by eating them with five almonds or a tablespoon of pumpkin seeds. Other than chestnuts, almonds are the best nut because they have the most protein compared with calories. Pumpkin seeds are also high in protein and in omega-3 fats.

Another snack option would be a bread, as listed below, with a protein-based spread. Cottage cheese, hummus and peanut butter are good examples. Hummus tastes great with oatcakes, on rye bread or with a raw carrot. (A large carrot is still less than 5GLs.) If you like peanut butter, buy the kind with no added sugar. Or you could have sugar-free beans on toast. A slice of any of the bread servings below with either hummus or peanut butter gives you the right kind of low-GL carbohydrate with some protein to keep your blood sugar level even.

Oatcakes, and oats in general, are excellent as far as weight and blood sugar are concerned. Of all the grains, oats are the best for losing weight, and for controlling your blood sugar.[5] Watch out when buying oatcakes, though. Many contain sugar. The best are Nairns since not only do they have sugar-free, organic types but they also use palm fruit oil, which contains unsaturated fat, as opposed to palm oil, which is higher in saturated fat.

Alternatively, have a bowl of low-GL soup made with vegetables and a protein element such as beans, lentils, nuts or chestnuts, or have a small salad of crunchy vegetables scattered with nuts and a little feta cheese, for example.

The GLs for bread and bread-substitute servings for snacks

Bread	5GLs
Oatcakes	2 biscuits
Rye 'pumpernickel' style	1 thin slice
Sourdough rye bread	1 thin slice
Rye wholemeal bread (yeasted)	half a slice
Wheat wholemeal bread (yeasted)	half a slice
White, high-fibre bread (yeasted)	less than half a slice (best avoided)

Here is a selection of 5GL snacks to choose from:

- A piece of fruit, plus five almonds or a tablespoon of pumpkin seeds.

- A thin slice of rye bread or two oatcakes and ½ small tub of cottage cheese (150g/5½oz).

- A thin slice of rye bread/two oatcakes and ½ small tub of hummus (150g/5½oz).

- A thin slice of rye bread/two oatcakes and peanut butter.

- Crudités (a carrot, pepper, cucumber or celery) and hummus.

- Crudités and cottage cheese.

- A small yoghurt (150g/5½oz), no sugar, plus berries; or cottage cheese plus berries.

As you can see, you won't be bored between meals, as there's plenty of scope for mixing and matching.

Simple ways to lower the GL of a meal

- Add a dash of lemon juice.
- Make it into a soup – it's more filling that way.
- Soak oats or eat them as porridge.
- Chew well and sip water.
- Put your fork down between mouthfuls.
- Add a dessertspoonful (two teaspoons) of oat bran (see page 215).
- Don't add sweet sauces.
- Wait 30 minutes before eating something sweet.
- Have dessert as a snack and include some protein.

For vegetarians

If you're a strict vegetarian, you'll need to eat more beans, lentils, soya produce (such as tofu and tempeh) and Quorn than usual to achieve the target for your protein intake. A serving size of tofu for a main meal is 160g (5¾oz), which is roughly three-quarters of a packet. Many recipes containing chicken or fish can be adapted by replacing them with tofu or a tofu steak.

What to have as a low-GL drink and eat for dessert

You have a daily 5GL allowance for drinks or desserts. A variety of drinks are possible within the 5GL rule:

The GLs in non-alcoholic drinks

Drink	5GLs
Tomato juice	600ml (20fl oz/1 pint)
Carrot juice	small glass
Grapefruit juice, unsweetened	small glass
Apple juice, unsweetened	small glass, diluted 50:50 with water
Orange juice, unsweetened	small glass, diluted 50:50 with water; or juice of one orange
Pineapple juice	half a small glass, diluted 50:50 with water
Cranberry juice drink	half a small glass, diluted 50:50 with water
Grape juice	an inch of liquid!

What about desserts? If you are used to eating a lot of desserts, or if you are insulin-resistant, you will probably crave something sweet at the end of each meal. It is very important to break this habit because if you don't it will keep your blood sugar level seesawing. It takes only three days in most cases to stop the craving. So, after your initial stimulant- and sugar-free period, limit desserts to one a week, perhaps at the weekend.

Don't have desserts when you are eating out, because almost all restaurant desserts are heavily loaded with sugar and saturated fat.

Accompaniment serving sizes

When it comes to knowing how much rice, pasta or potatoes to serve with your meals, you can vary the portion according to whether you want to stick to the 45GLs per day weight-loss limit, or relax this a bit to 65GLs to maintain weight. There is a handy reference guide on page 228 to show you roughly how much of each of the healthiest carbohydrate choices you could eat.

Food	7GLs approximate serving (for weight loss)	10GLs approximate serving (for heart health and weight maintenance)
Brown basmati rice (dried)	40g (1½oz)	60g (2⅓oz)
Wholemeal pasta (dried)	40g (1½oz)	55g (2oz)
Quinoa (dried)	65g (2¼oz)	95g (3¼oz) (NB very large serving)
Baked potato/sweet potato	½	1 small
Boiled baby new potatoes	75g (2¾oz) (approximately 3)	125g (4½oz) (approximately 4)
Beans, pulses (approximate value; different types can vary)	½ a 410g (14½oz) can	¾ a 410g (14½oz) can
Rough milled oatcakes	4	5–6
Rye bread (e.g. pumpernickel or sourdough)	1 slice is 10GLs	1 slice
Wholemeal wheaten bread	1 slice is 10GLs	1 slice

The right fats and oils

This diet is not low fat. In fact the aim is to ensure that you regularly eat the correct balance of essential omega-3 fats while limiting harmful trans-fats and saturated fats.

As far as fats and oils go, what's important is which fats you use, and how you use them.

Creams If you want to make a savoury dish creamier, try adding a teaspoon of tahini (sesame spread) or a tablespoon of coconut milk or coconut cream.

Salad dressings When using seed oils for salad dressings, pick either flaxseed oil or a blend of oils that gives at least one part omega-3 fats to one part of omega-6 fats. These seed oils need to be cold-pressed and stored in a lightproof container.

A good seed oil blend is Udo's Choice, available in health-food stores (see Resources). Also good is walnut oil or a virgin pressed organic olive oil. You can lightly drizzle these oils onto vegetables instead of butter.

Cooking oils For steam-frying (see below) and sautéing, use a small amount of butter, coconut butter or olive oil. Coconut butter adds a great flavour to steam-fries.

Quick planning and tasty cooking

Although it is easy to make healthy meals following the guidelines above, if you prefer to follow recipes you will find *The 10 Secrets of 100% Health Cookbook* by myself and Fiona McDonald Joyce helpful and inspiring. It contains delicious low-GL recipes and a chart to help you map out your week's menus to ensure you have sufficient levels of omega-3 oils, B vitamins and ORACs. Here is a taster:

Symbols
The recipes with the most Ω have the most omega-3s.
Those with the most * have the most antioxidants.
Those with the most B have the most homocysteine-lowering B vitamins.
The GL score is also given.

Meal	Recipe	GLs	Essential fats	ORACs	B vitamins
Day 1					
Breakfast	Poached eggs on soda bread	6	ΩΩΩ	–	B
Snack	A small plain yoghurt plus ½ punnet berries	5	–	******	BB
Lunch	Kedgeree with green salad	8	ΩΩ	****	BBB
Snack	3 oatcakes and ½ small tub of cottage cheese	6	–	–	B
Dinner	Chicken and Puy lentil stew with new potatoes and steamed broccoli	15	–	******	BBB
Drinks/ dessert	Optional – of your choice but no more than 5GLs	5			
Total		45	ΩΩΩΩΩ	*************	BBBBB BBBB

Day 2					
Breakfast	Porridge with almonds and goji	3	–	*	B
Snack	Crudités and hummus	5	–	****	BB
Lunch	Smoked salmon stuffed avocado with chia loaf	10	ΩΩΩ	****	BBB
Snack	Fresh fruit and 2 tbsp pumpkin seeds	7	Ω	****	BB
Dinner	Tofu noodle stir fry	15	–	*	BBB
Drinks/ dessert	Optional – of your choice but no more than 5GLs	5			
Total		**45**	ΩΩΩΩ	******* *******	BBBBB BBBBB

Cooking methods

All carbohydrate foods release their carbohydrate somewhat faster once cooked. The longer you cook something and the higher the temperature, the faster releasing the food becomes. It's therefore best to eat food as close to raw as possible. Also 'wet' cooking methods, such as steaming, generate fewer oxidants than dry cooking, such as baking.[6] Crisps are especially bad news in this respect.

This doesn't mean eating endless salads. You can steam, steam-fry, boil and poach food without cooking it to death. Next best is baking, grilling, sautéing or stir-frying. Worst is frying or deep-frying.

Steaming is the best way to cook green, leafy, less starchy vegetables, since it preserves a lot of their vitamins and minimises any raising of GL. This method can be used with any food and is very success-ful with fish – but perhaps not ideal with starchy vegetables, which require longer cooking, or with red meat. Many different kinds of steamers are available, or you can improvise with a colander, pan and lid.

Boiling raises the GL of foods more than steaming, but less than bak-ing. Changes can be kept to a minimum by using as little water as

possible, keeping the lid on, and cooking the food as whole as possible. Also, eat all vegetables al dente – a little crisp, not soft.

Steam-frying adds loads of taste without compromising on health.
The great advantage of this style of cooking is that the lower temperature of steaming doesn't destroy nutrients to anything like the extent
that frying does, and you use only a small amount of oil, if that. As
with boiling and ordinary steaming, aim to keep vegetables al dente.

To steam-fry, use a shallow pan or a deep frying pan with a thick
base and lid that seals well. You can steam-fry without oil by first
adding two tablespoons of liquid to the pan – water, vegetable stock,
soy sauce or some watered-down sauce you'll use for the dish. Once
it boils, immediately add some vegetables, sauté rapidly for a minute
or two, turn the heat up, add a tablespoon or two more of the liquid
and clamp the lid on tightly. After a minute add the remaining ingredients. Turn the heat down after a couple of minutes and steam in
this way until cooked.

Or you can add a teaspoon to a tablespoon of olive oil, butter or
coconut oil to the pan, warm it, add the ingredients and sauté. After a
couple of minutes, add two tablespoons of liquid as above and clamp
the lid on. Steam the ingredients until done.

Poaching is like steam-frying without the sautéing. You can make
delicious water-based sauces; for example, you could cook fish in
vegetable broth flavoured with ginger, garlic, lemongrass, spices and
wine (the alcohol boils off).

Waterless cooking requires specially designed pans in which you can
'boil' foods by steaming them in their own juice and 'fry' foods with no
oil. Both methods are excellent for preserving nutrients and flavour.

Baking is useful, especially if the food is large and has a thick skin
(such as a whole or half squash or pumpkin). Avoid coating food
with oil, because the oil will oxidise with cooking, which creates free
radicals (highly reactive, harmful molecules). You can roast a potato
without adding oil. The higher the temperature and the longer you
cook something, the higher the GL becomes.

Frying should be kept to a minimum, and deep-frying avoided altogether. When you do fry use butter, coconut oil (saturated fat) or olive oil (monounsaturated) rather than other vegetable oils (poly-unsaturated oils), since these are much more prone to oxidation.

Grilling foods that contain fat is less damaging than frying, but browning or burning food does create free radicals. Try to avoid bar-becued food, or at least ensure that what you eat is not charred.

Microwaving is a problematic cooking method, although admittedly fast. As food cooks in its own water, it seems better than most cooking methods for preserving the water-soluble vitamins B and C; how-ever, the temperatures reached in fat particles are very high, so avoid microwaving oily fish as this will destroy the essential fats it contains. And remember that microwave ovens do give off electromagnetic radiation, even 1.8m (6ft) away. It is better to use lower-voltage/heat settings for longer cooking. Cover dishes to encourage steaming, although you do need to leave some room for steam to escape.

Fill yourself up with the good stuff

Low-GL eating isn't difficult once you get the hang of it. You can also apply the principles quite easily when you eat out, choosing smaller carb portions, perhaps sharing rice or potatoes with your friend, and having more vegetable 'side' dishes. It is also very filling and that's the key. Fill yourself up with the good stuff, then your desire for the kind of foods that got you into trouble in the first place will recede.

If you'd like more support in following my low-GL diet you can join a Zest4Life group in your area (see Resources). There are also a variety of cookbooks using my low-GL diet: *The Low-GL Diet Cookbook*, *The 10 Secrets of 100% Health Cookbook* and *Food GLorious Food*, which gives you delicious low-GL recipes from around the world. Soon you will discover that this way of eating becomes your way of life.

CHAPTER 22

Essential Supplements

Throughout this book you will have seen copious evidence of the value of specific doses of nutrients both to prevent and to aid rapid recovery from heart disease. Despite this evidence you will still encounter intelligent but ill-informed experts who say that supplements are a waste of time, and they might even try to dissuade you from taking them out of a fear of side effects. In more than 30 years of clinical experience I have yet to witness such side effects and, conversely, have seen many people make significant health transformations through the combination of diet and optimal supplementation.

Even basic multivitamins make a difference. A survey in Sweden of over 30,000 women found that those taking a daily multivitamin for five years or more reduced their risk of having a heart attack by 41 per cent; however, among those who already had cardiovascular disease simply taking a multivitamin didn't reduce risk.[7] The moral of this story is that you need much more than a multivitamin to reverse heart disease. You need to pull out all the stops.

Almost always the optimal level of a nutrient to help bring your system back into balance is far greater than what you need to maintain health. This is clear from the research, and is also a fundamental principle of nutritional medicine. Nutrients, in large amounts, do correct underlying disease processes.

On page 234 I list the nutrients that the research shows have the effects of lowering blood pressure, improving cholesterol ratios, improving heart-muscle function and supporting cardiovascular health.

The dosages of nutrients for cardiovascular health

Nutrient	Daily Dosage
Niacin	1,000–2,000mg
Folic acid	400–800mcg
Vitamin B_{12}	250–500mcg
Vitamin B_6	20–50mg
TMG	500–1,000mg
Magnesium	300mg
Omega-3 fish oil	2,000mg
Vitamin E	100–500mg
CoQ_{10}	30–120mg
Carnitine	500–2,000mg

Your supplement programme should include at least the lower levels of these nutrients.

Building your own perfect supplement programme depends on which critical health factors discussed in Part 2 relate to you. Also, if you have high blood pressure, high cholesterol or angina, or if you are recovering from a heart attack or stroke, the chapters in Part 3 will give you guidance on which key nutrient strategies to focus on.

Many of these nutrients are available combined in specific supplement formulas. In practical terms, a typical supplement programme to prevent or reverse cardiovascular disease might look like this (the basic supplements are in bold):

- **High-strength multivitamin twice a day**

- **Vitamin C 1,000mg twice a day**

- **Omega-3 fish oil once** or twice a day

- Non-blushing niacin 500mg once or twice a day

- Antioxidant complex once or twice a day

- CoQ_{10} 30mg with l-carnitine one to four times a day

- Homocysteine-lowering formula one to three times a day (if homocysteine is high)

You won't necessarily need all of these unless you are going for full-on recovery. What you need depends on your circumstances, but whatever your circumstances I'd always start with the basics, shown in bold above.

The basics

There are three basic supplements, the foundation of any good supplement programme, that are recommended for everybody with or without cardiovascular disease. These are:

- A high-strength, 'optimum nutrition' multivitamin–mineral

- Extra vitamin C plus other immune-boosting nutrients – a vitamin C 1g complex

- An essential omega-3 and -6 supplement (you need ten times more omega-3 than omega-6)

I take these every day and I recommend you do the same. But how do you know which formulations to choose?

The best multis

Any decent multivitamin and mineral will tell you to take two a day, preferably one at breakfast and one at lunch, firstly because you cannot get enough of all the nutrients in one pill, and secondly because the water-soluble vitamins B and C are in and out of your body in four to six hours, so you get twice the benefit by taking them twice a day. Many multivitamins skimp on the minerals. A hallmark of a good one is that it will provide at least 150mg of magnesium, 10mg of zinc, plus 25mcg of selenium and chromium. Another hallmark of a good multivitamin is its vitamin D content. You need at least 15mcg a day. Also vitamin E – a good multi should provide around 100mg. I call this a high-strength or 'optimum nutrition' multivitamin, so that it is not confused with the very basic, and rather ineffective, RDA-level multis.

The best vitamin C supplements

The form of vitamin C itself doesn't make as much difference as people make out. Ascorbic acid, ascorbate, 'ester' C – they all work. But there are other nutrients and herbs that support health and immunity. These include zinc, black elderberry extracts and anthocyanidins (for example, found in bilberry). So a vitamin C supplement that also contains these synergistic ingredients gives you more bang for your buck. Ideally you want something like 2,000mg of vitamin C in total a day, but you can get 200mg if you eat six or more servings of the right fruit and vegetables a day. So that leaves 1,800mg – or 900mg twice a day. That's a good level for general health maintenance. Vitamin C products that contain significant amounts of anthocyanidins will have a purple hue. I call this a vitamin C 1g complex.

The best essential-fat supplements

The most potent forms of omega-3 are called EPA, DPA and DHA. These are found in oily fish. The most potent omega-6 is called GLA. This is found in borage and evening primrose oil. Since we need more, and are more deficient in, omega-3, you need at least ten times more omega-3 than -6. (Add up the total EPA, DPA and DHA in a supplement and divide by the total GLA. This figure should be over 10.) In all you are looking for at least 600mg of combined EPA, DPA and DHA a day for general health maintenance. It is not worth supplementing the vegetarian form of omega-3, alpha-linolenic acid, such as linseed oil capsules, as you can get this from eating seeds together with fibre. I call this an essential omega supplement. If you have cardiovascular disease, you may also need to top up extra EPA from a concentrated fish oil source. These are usually called something like omega EPA.

Optional extras

Vitamin D If your multi doesn't provide 15mcg of vitamin D, you need to supplement this. During winter it's ideal to have 25–50mcg a day, which is one or two 1000iu vitamin D drops a day.

Homocysteine-lowering B vitamins (depending on your homo-cysteine levels). If you have elevated homocysteine, look for a homocysteine-lowering formulation which ideally contains vitamins B_6 (50mg), B_{12} (500mcg), folic acid (800mg), B_2 and the mineral zinc along with TMG (1,000mg) and NAC. Use the chart below to work out how much you need depending on your homocysteine level.

If your H score is below 6, you can achieve these kinds of levels from a high-strength multivitamin; however, if your score is above 6 you will need to also take a specific supplement containing all these nutrients, designed to normalise your homocysteine level.

Homocysteine level

Nutrient Hcy score	No risk below 7	Low risk 7–9	At risk 10–15	High risk above 15
Folate	200mcg	400mcg	800mcg	800mcg
B_{12}	10mcg	250mcg	500mcg	750mcg
B_6	10mg	20mg	25mg	50mg
B_2	5mg	10mg	15mg	25mg
Zinc	5mg	10mg	15mg	20mg
TMG	–	500mg	750mg	1500mg
NAC	–	250mg	500mg	750mg

Niacin If you have raised lipoprotein(a), LDL cholesterol or triglycerides, or low HDL cholesterol, then the most effective treatment is not statins, but niacin, which is available on prescription. Otherwise you can take non-blushing forms of niacin (but not niacinamide – also known as nicotinamide – which doesn't work) or the blushing form of niacin, nicotinic acid (also known as nicotinate), 500mg twice a day. (Not everybody tolerates the blushing form well, but the blushing reduces after a few days and is less pronounced if taken with a meal.)

Antioxidant complex Look for formulas that provide: glutathione or n-acetyl cysteine (NAC), alpha-lipoic acid, vitamin E, vitamin C (not so essential since it appears in the basics), CoQ_{10}, resveratrol, anthocyanidins, carotenoids and vitamin A. I take one of these anti-oxidant complexes every day. Take up to three if you are recovering from cardiovascular disease or a recent event.

Vitamin C I recommend everyone takes 900mg twice a day. If you have high cholesterol or high blood pressure take 1g three times a day; if you have angina or atherosclerosis take 2g three times a day.

Lysine If you have atherosclerosis or angina, take 1g of lysine three times a day.

CoQ$_{10}$ There's a good case for taking 30mg of CoQ$_{10}$ every day for prevention. Take 90mg a day if on statins and 120mg a day divided into four doses if recovering from a cardiovascular event or if you have poor heart function. (Speak to your doctor if you are on blood-thinning medication.)

    Carnitine is best taken with CoQ$_{10}$ in a formula containing propionyl-L-carnitine. Take 250mg of carnitine with every 60mg of CoQ$_{10}$.

Magnesium Anyone with cardiovascular concerns should supplement 300mg magnesium a day. A good multivitamin might provide 150mg, leaving an additional 150mg daily. Some high-dose niacin formulas contain extra magnesium which, together with a good multivitamin, might give you the needed 300mg a day. Otherwise, you'll need to take a magnesium supplement. Magnesium ascorbate is available as a powder, giving you both vitamin C and magnesium.

L-arginine taken in the dose range of 2,000–3,000mg along with **L-citrulline** 200–300mg, taken twice a day, supports nitric oxide (NO) production.

Phosphatidyl or cdp choline If you are recovering from a stroke, also take either 3 teaspoons of hi-phosphatidyl lecithin granules, sprinkled on food, or 500mg of cdp choline or six lecithin capsules a day.

This is the 'palette' of potential supplements. Which ones you need depends on both your key areas of weakness, as discussed in Part 2, backed up by your test results, and your current cardiovascular health.

Weight support

If you are overweight, losing weight needs to be a priority for restoring cardiovascular health.

Glucomannan and PGX Along with a strict low-GL diet the superfibres glucomannan and PGX, available as a supplemental powder or capsules taken before meals, will fill you up and lower the GL of your meal. These are worth considering if you need to lose weight. Aim for 3–5g (a teaspoonful) before each main meal.

Chromium and cinnamon extract also help to stabilise blood sugar and improve insulin sensitivity.

Getting help

If you are recovering from a cardiovascular event or are on medication for heart disease, I recommend you book a consultation with a nutritional therapist who can help get you started on the right supplement programme for you (see Resources to find one near you). They can help you through the maze and give you combination supplements that will mean that you can take fewer actual pills.

Do check with your doctor that there is nothing you intend to take that is contra-indicated with medication. If your doctor is switched on, they'll be pleased you are taking a pro-active approach and will want to monitor your progress with a view to reducing medication.

IMPORTANT Don't change your medication without consulting your doctor.

The amount of supplements you need to take will also reduce in time. If you are perfectly healthy, just take the basics. In my fifties, with optimal cardiovascular health, I take a high-strength multivitamin, essential omegas and vitamin C twice a day, and an antioxidant and phospholipid complex once a day, most days.

CHAPTER 23

How to Exercise Your Heart

To avoid developing heart disease, or to help reverse it, you need to build exercise into your weekly routine, as I have explained in Chapter 15. The combination of an optimal diet (my Heart-friendly Diet) and optimal exercise is a winning formula. According to a comprehensive review in the journal *Circulation*, simply taking 30 minutes or more of moderate-intensity activity on most days could cut your risk of a fatal heart attack by a quarter.[8] What is more, this doesn't have to be all in one go, so you could walk to the shops (15 minutes), then spend 15 minutes doing something active at home, be it gardening or cleaning the house. All of this makes a difference depending on how you do it. By simply building exercise into your life you will help to prevent atherosclerosis and coronary artery disease, reduce triglyceride levels, raise HDL and lower blood pressure,[9] as well as burning fat and stabilising your blood sugar levels, all of which are exceedingly good news for your heart and arteries.

NOTE Before starting your exercise regime, don't forget to check with your doctor, and remember to start off gently and build up as you get fitter, especially if you've had some damage to your heart or currently have angina. If you join an exercise class of any kind the trainer will advise you how to begin. The advantage of an exercise class is that, contrary to what you might believe, most people are not super-fit but just ordinary people of all fitness levels working hard to improve their fitness, and the classes are often very friendly.

Why take aerobic exercise?

You may remember from Chapter 15 that I described aerobic exercise as long and steady to build up heart strength. To improve glycemic control, assist with weight maintenance, and reduce your risk of cardiovascular disease, I recommend at least 150 minutes per week of moderate-intensity aerobic physical activity (meaning within your training heart-rate zone, see page 242).

The physical activity should be distributed over at least three days per week and with no more than two consecutive days without physical activity.

Even better than the above is doing slightly shorter sessions, maybe with high-intensity exercises, three times a week, but you'll need to follow the guidance of a fitness instructor if you have heart disease.

Why do you need resistance exercise?

For cardiovascular health you also need to build and maintain muscle strength throughout the body and this is achieved through resistance exercise. Resistance exercise means exercising against some force (such as weights, springs or an exercise band) so that muscle can be built up. This could also involve simple exercises such as slow sit-ups or Pilates, which also build muscle. Ideally, you should be doing some kind of resistance exercise three times a week, strengthening all the major muscle groups. If you are recovering from a cardiovascular event you'll be advised to build up slowly to this goal.

These two kinds of exercise, aerobic and resistance, have two different effects. You can think of them as the difference between a long-distance runner and a sprinter. The long-distance runner is lean, while the sprinter has more muscle. The ideal is a bit of both, because you are aiming to burn fat, and when you build muscle you naturally raise the growth hormone, which helps to improve insulin sensitivity as well as giving you more muscle to burn more fat. All this will normalise your cholesterol and triglyceride levels.

The type of exercise is as important as the duration

If you are doing the right kind of exercise (that is, a mixture of aerobic and resistance), all you need to do is 20–30 minutes a day. And this will be enough both for losing weight, if you need to, and helping to reverse heart disease. If you want to confine your exercising to five days a week, you can do 30 minutes a day with two days off. If you are doing less strenuous exercise you may need to increase your daily time of exercising to 30–45 minutes a day, but it is important to build up the intensity. My advice is to make an appointment in your diary to exercise, just like you would to attend a meeting or see a friend. Then, don't break it.

What kind of aerobic exercise could you take?

Depending on your current level of fitness, aerobic exercise can be anything from brisk walking to playing golf, going for a swim or a bike ride or joining an exercise class, or even just being more active at home, climbing the stairs, gardening or vacuum cleaning, but the key is that you get your heart rate into your 'training heart-rate zone'.

Your training heart-rate zone

To find your training heart-rate zone, you need to subtract your age from 220, then calculate 65 per cent of this amount for the lower end of your training zone and 80 per cent for the upper limit:

220 – [age] × .65 = lower limit
220 – [age] × .80 = upper limit

For example, for a 50-year-old:

220 – 50 = 170 × .65 = lower limit = 110 beats per minute
220 – 50 = 170 × .80 = upper limit = 136 beats per minute

You should be exercising for at least 15 minutes with your pulse in this training heart-rate zone. If you measure your pulse for 10 seconds, then multiply it by 6, you'll find out if you are exercising hard enough, or too hard.

An overweight, out-of-condition person may reach their training heart-rate zone by walking just a few hundred yards. A fitter, leaner person may have to walk briskly for at least five minutes to push their pulse up to their training zone. This is why you need to monitor your pulse while exercising to make sure you do not over- or under-exercise, and to achieve the best benefits for burning fat and to strengthen your heart. As you get fitter and leaner, you'll find that you will have to push harder – perhaps by walking faster or adding more hill walking to your programme – to reach your training zone.

What kind of resistance exercise gives the best results?

Resistance exercise is akin to building muscle, but you don't need to be lifting a whole ton of weight to do this! To understand why this type of exercise is important it's good to know that there are three different kinds of muscle fibres and, ideally, you want more of all three. These are:

1   Slow (red muscle, which contains more oxygen)

2   Fast (white muscle)

3   Super-fast (white muscle)

Your aerobic exercise is working mainly the slow muscle. When you work the fast or, even better, the super-fast muscle – for example in a sprint – this is beyond your oxygen capacity and is called 'anaerobic' exercise. At the end you'll be puffing and panting.

Why high-intensity exercise works well

The interesting thing is that if you do the right kind of high-intensity exercise – using and developing super-fast muscle – you don't need to do it for long. It can literally be a 30-second burst of intense exercise, five to eight times. That's it. Do this three times a week and you'll get a great result. It makes your heart muscle work hard, so you'll be really panting at the end of your 30 seconds, and this can increase your growth hormone level by up to five times, which then both re-sensitises you to insulin, and builds muscle.

One of the original proponents of this type of exercising is Phil Campbell, author of *Ready, Set, Go!* (see Recommended Reading), which is a great book to read if you want to go into this in more detail. He's a trainer of top athletes and sportsmen, but don't be put off by that – the principles are really simple. You can see for yourself by watching the YouTube video made by Dr Joseph Mercola, who describes a version of these principles as the Peak 8 system (see Resources). This is based on eight sprints, in this case done on an exercise bike, but you can do it with any kind of exercise – sprinting, swimming or cycling, for example. The basic guidelines are as follows:

1 You warm up for three minutes.

2 Now exercise as hard and fast as you can for 30 seconds. You should feel like you couldn't possibly go on for another few seconds.

3 Recover for 90 seconds.

4 Then do it again.

5 Repeat this cycle a total of eight times.

That's the goal, but Rome wasn't built in a day, and it is really important to build up to this if you are currently not in good shape. That might mean doing the sequence only two or three times first time, then adding a repetition as you become more able.

At the first level, for example, you might be walking for three minutes, then have a 30-second burst of walking or jogging as fast as you can, then you stop. You want to get your heart rate up into the top end of your training heart-rate zone.

You know you've reached it when it's hard to breathe and talk due to the temporary oxygen debt; you start to sweat; you feel hot; and you get some muscle ache. But simply doing this three times a week will make a big difference to your health, building muscle, burning fat and helping restore blood sugar control. This whole sequence takes 20 minutes. Peak 8 builds muscles in your abdomen, bottom, legs, chest and shoulders.

If you have angina or have had a heart attack or stroke you must be guided by your doctor as to the level of exercise that you can take and build up to your training heart-rate zone very gradually – perhaps over a period of weeks or months. Remember that simply exercising will bring benefits and that trying to aim for too much too soon will put a strain on your heart; your heart's strength needs to be built up slowly.

Toning and building muscle in other ways

Other forms of resistance exercise include using weights, bands or springs, practising Pilates or yoga, and by simple exercises like squats and sit-ups that you can do at home. A simple routine is shown on my website www.holforddiet.com under 'fatburning exercises'. Ideally choose a selection that works both your upper and lower body muscles.

Your weekly routine

Choose the kind of training that appeals to you, making sure that the aerobic exercise will raise your heart rate into the training zone. Don't try to do too much to start with, especially if you have any degree of angina or a weaker heart. If you are very unfit or overweight it is essential to get some professional guidance and support at the beginning. Now plan your week ahead. A typical weekly routine might look like this, but you will need to build up to it if you are very unfit:

Monday – resistance training (20 minutes)
Tuesday – aerobic exercise (30-plus minutes)
Wednesday – resistance training (20 minutes)
Thursday – aerobic exercise (30-plus minutes)
Friday – resistance training (20 minutes)
Saturday – aerobic exercise (30 minutes)
Sunday – day off

If you are working with a fitness instructor, make sure he or she includes both aerobic and resistance training. You are aiming to exercise for at least 150 minutes a week, or 20–30 minutes every day, or 30 minutes five times a week.

When is the best time to exercise?

The best time to exercise is two hours after eating. No self-respecting animal would eat before exercising. From an evolutionary perspective the purpose of exercise is to get food to eat. If you exercise first thing in the morning, make sure you have breakfast straight after. When you eat after exercising, your muscles and liver are geared up to deal with the carbohydrates in your food so you don't get such big spikes in your blood sugar.

Having said that, going for a stroll after a main meal – for example after Sunday lunch – then having your dessert after the walk also helps to stabilise blood sugar levels.

Don't exercise late at night. Also, if possible, exercise in natural daylight because you'll make vitamin D, which strengthens bones.

Warm up before aerobic exercise by starting off slowly, and before resistance exercises warm up by walking or stretching.

Increasing your daily activity level

Of course, you don't have to join a gym and start a training regime to gain health improvements. Another way of looking at it is in terms of physical activity. Do you spend most of your day sitting at a desk? Do you take the lift and never use the stairs? Does a trip to the supermarket always involve a car ride? Are escalators only meant for standing on? Although there are a multitude of ways to increase your daily activity levels, what we really need is a simple way of assessing activity, and this is where the term METs comes into play.

One MET – or metabolic unit of energy – equals the amount of energy spent when you are totally at rest, perhaps sitting in a chair or lying down in bed. The moment you start moving, your heart rate increases, you breathe more deeply and you expend energy. A simple calculation based on maximum heart rate and maximum breathing rate makes it possible to measure the physical activity or level of effort required for any human activity in METs. So 2 METS is twice the effort of 1 MET. How can we relate this value to everyday actions?

In the following table you'll find a list of everyday activities and their MET ratings. If you consider that the recommended level of daily exercise is a brisk 30–40-minute walk at 5–6km (3–3¾ miles) per hour, and that this uses 5–6 METs, you can see the relative value of any other activity. So, if you don't go out for your jog, the equivalent activity would be gardening or heavier housework for the same length of time. Just add up all your activities and you'll see how much (or how little!) you move in a day. If you switched from doing moderate housekeeping to mowing the lawn you would double your METS.

The METs for various activities

1 MET	Sleeping	Lying in bed
	Sitting in a chair	
2 METs	Standing	Talking
	Walking (1.6km (1 mile)/h)	Reading
	Shaving	Writing
	Playing cards	Light housekeeping
	Typing	(dusting)
	Brushing hair	

2–3 METs	Walking (3.2 km (2 miles)/h)	Washing hair
	Bathing	Playing piano
	Moderate housekeeping (light laundry)	Cycling (8km (5 miles)/h)
3–4 METs	Walking (5km (3 miles)/h)	Cycling (13km (8 miles)/h)
	Climbing stairs slowly	Heavier housework (scrubbing dishes)
4–5 METS	Walking (6.5km (4 miles)/h)	Cycling (14km (8½miles)/h)
	Heavy housework (vacuum cleaning)	Mowing lawn (power)
		Gardening
	Playing badminton/tennis	Washing windows
5–6 METs	Walking (7.2km (4½)/h)	Cycling (16km (10 miles)/h)
	Light shovelling	Golfing
	Heavy housework (scrubbing floors)	Carrying groceries
6–7 METs	Walking (8km (5 miles)/h)	Cycling (18km (11¼ miles)/h)
	Leisurely swim	Moving furniture
	Mowing lawn (push mower)	Playing tennis (singles)
7–8 METs	Jogging (8km (5 miles)/h)	Cycling (19.5km (12 miles)/h)
	Swimming laps (slowly)	Climbing stairs
	Playing football	Playing tennis (competitive singles)
8–9 METs	Jogging (9km (5½ miles)/h)	Cycling (21km (13 miles)/h)
	Swimming laps (fast)	Carrying groceries upstairs
	Playing basketball	Cross-country skiing
10+ METs	Handball, squash	Jogging (10km (6¼ miles)/h)
	Climbing hills with a load	

Your goal is to get up to the 5–6 METs range. If you currently have less than a 3-MET capacity, it's best to engage in multiple short daily exercise sessions. If you are in the 3–5 MET range you have the capacity to do 1–2 exercise sessions a day. If you are already in the 5-MET-plus category, make sure you maintain your activity with 3–5 exercise sessions a week.

As you can see from the chart on page 249, a great way to increase your general level of exercise is simply to get more active generally.

Use the stairs instead of the lift. Walk or cycle instead of driving everywhere. Run around with your kids or grandchildren, or take up a sport. There are many opportunities in a day to develop fitness, and soon this way of living will become a habit.

Get fit by taking the alternative way

The fat way	**The fit way**
Take a lift	Use the stairs
Use a trolley when shopping	Use a hand basket
Drive to work	Walk or cycle some of the way
Drive to the shops	Walk to the shops
Spend the night watching TV	Take up an active hobby
Get other people to bring you one too	Get up and do it yourself
Use powered tools for gardening or DIY work	Use manual tools when it's just as quick
Go upstairs as little as possible at home	Run upstairs as often as possible
Use automatic car washes	Wash the car yourself
Stick the children in front of the TV	Actively play with them
Have business meetings inside	Go for a walk where possible

CHAPTER 24

How to Live a Low-stress Life

As you saw in Chapter 9, stress is a major risk factor for heart disease, high blood pressure and high cholesterol. When you feel stressed, your body is preparing you for 'fight or flight'. Unlike the past, when our ancestors were hunting for food or encountering wild animals, and stress helped them to react extremely quickly, 'fight' to modern people means you feel irritable, aggressive and stressed out, while 'flight' means you feel anxious and want to run away, feeling trapped in your circumstances. Do you ever feel like this?

Many people live in a state of anxiety. They arrive at work stressed out from commuting, then they have to contend with a lot of stress at work. By the time they go home they are in a state of near collapse.

How stressed are you?

Take a look at the symptoms below. If they sound familiar to you, then you'll know what I'm talking about:

- Do you have difficulty getting up in the morning?

- Are you tired all the time?

- Do you crave certain foods?

- Do you feel anger, irritability or aggressiveness?

- Do you have mood swings?

- Are you restless?

- Do you have an energy slump during the day?

- Do you have regular feelings of weakness?

- Do you feel apathy?

- Are you depressed?

- Do you feel cold a lot of the time?

The above symptoms suggest adrenal stress overload. Most people report that they experience a high number of these kinds of symptoms. In the 100% Health Survey, 82 per cent of respondents said that they easily became impatient, 81 per cent said they had low energy, 68 per cent said they felt they had too much to do, and 66 per cent said they became anxious or tense easily.[10]

The dangers of too much stress and cortisol

With long-term stress, the adrenal hormone cortisol stays high. Meanwhile, the circulating levels of three chemicals that help you to relax decline – these are GABA, which switches off adrenalin; serotonin, which keeps you happy; and DHEA, the revitalising hormone. Your mood gets worse, your sleep gets worse, you have more and more blood sugar spikes and troughs, and you produce more and more insulin as insulin resistance sets in.

Whenever your blood sugar level crashes, the body produces yet more cortisol. It thinks you are being starved and so it goes into panic mode. Your brain is literally working overtime and demanding more sugar so that your blood sugar levels stay high.[11]

If you think about it, in a real state of emergency, certainly one where you are taking physical action, the last thing you want to do is eat. Your whole body gears up to liberate its stores of energy so that you can react quickly to the emergency. When you are really pumped up, stress acts as an appetite suppressant.

Continued stress messes this up. Rather than not eating at all, many people find that they compulsively eat – and they eat all the wrong things, such as sugary foods. This is a recipe for disaster, because now you have cortisol trying to raise your blood sugar level, and interfering with insulin, and you have your blood sugar level rising from what you've eaten, telling your body to make more insulin. You end up with high blood glucose, high blood pressure, high cholesterol and insulin resistance. This is the fast track to heart disease. By the way, people under stress also gravitate towards more salt. This is another sign of adrenal overload.

How a low-GL diet helps you to cope with life's difficulties

The amazing thing is that if you balance your blood sugar by following my low-GL Heart-friendly Diet and take the recommended supplements, it not only affects your weight and your heart but it also has wide-reaching benefits for your health, your mood and your ability to deal with the inevitable challenges of life. When you're stressed, even molehills seem like mountains.

When your energy levels are good and your mind is clear, life immediately smoothes out and calms down. People on my low-GL diet often report big improvements in mood, concentration and memory. In an eight-week trial we ran with volunteers on the Holford Diet, almost all (94 per cent) reported greater energy, two-thirds had greater concentration, memory or alertness, and half reported fewer feelings of depression and had more stable moods.[12]

The way back from stress

The only way out of the prison of stress, sugar and stimulants is:

1   To reduce or avoid all forms of concentrated sweetness, tea, coffee, alcohol and cigarettes, and to start eating foods that help

to keep your blood sugar level stable. By changing to the right foods, backed up with specific nutritional supplements, most people feel an amazing improvement in energy within days. It is especially important not to eat sweet foods when you feel stressed.

2   To learn how to maintain a calmer state of openness and positivity. (More on this in a minute.)

3   To exercise regularly, which is a biochemical, physiological and psychological antidote to stress, as I explained in the previous chapter.

Of course, it's easy to say 'reduce your stress level' but not so easy to do it – unless you know how. You might say that your stresses are beyond your control – the mortgage, debts, family problems, and so on. To some extent, this is true because changing your external circumstances can definitely reduce stress. A common source of stress, for example, is having unfinished business; to avoid feeling trapped by this overload, if you have too many commitments or things to complete, try to find a way to share your load, and don't take on new projects until you finish old ones. Also, learn to say no.

There are also other ways to deal with stress. Some people appear to stay calm most of the time, even when the pressure is on. How do they do this? Often we hear advice to meditate, practise yoga, breathe deeply, and so on, but when you are tired and over-stressed these things are not easy to do.

Reduce your stress by becoming 'coherent'

In Chapter 9 I mentioned a technique called HeartMath that can help you switch out of a stress reaction in difficult moments in a matter of seconds. HeartMath was devised by Doc Childre and Rollin McCraty, from the HeartMath Institute in California, who have spent the last decade studying exactly what happens in the different emotional states we move between.

Developing a positive attitude is key. In fact, the most dangerous emotion for both physical and psychological health is not depression but cynicism. Cynicism raises 'inflammatory markers' in the body, and the more cynical a person is the more those markers are raised. A study of people with atherosclerosis showed that being stressed was worse than being depressed, but the worst of all was being cynical.[13]

We often think the opposite of stress is relaxation – being in a calm, quiet state. But what Childre and McCraty discovered is that countering the unhealthy effects of stress is not just about calming down but about activating a positive emotional state.

HeartMath can teach you a simple technique that can be practised daily to help you actively reduce the stress in your life. The premise of HeartMath is different from many other approaches for relieving stress, which typically focus on calming down after the stressful event has occurred; for example, by going for a massage or having a glass of wine after a difficult day at work (although there's nothing wrong with this).

With HeartMath, you learn a simple breathing technique that can help you to 'reset' your physiological reaction to stress as the event occurs. Just a couple of HeartMath breaths can help you stop the cascade that triggers the release of cortisol. In doing so, you stay coherent (that is, calm and in balance). Research has found that exercise, when practised regularly, can help you to feel better emotionally and improve your intuition, creativity and cognitive performance.[14]

Here's a simple HeartMath exercise called the Quick Coherence Technique:

1 Heart focus Focus your attention on your heart area – the space behind your breastbone in the centre of your chest between your nipples (your heart is more in the centre than on the left).

2 Heart breathing Now imagine your breath flowing in and out of your heart area. This helps your respiration and heart rhythm to synchronise. Focus on this area and aim to breathe evenly; for example, inhale for five or six seconds and exhale for five or six seconds (choose a timescale that feels comfortable for you and flows easily).

3 Heart feeling As you breathe in and out of your heart area, recall a positive emotion and try to re-experience it. This could be remembering a time spent with someone you love, walking in your favourite spot, stroking a pet, picturing a tree you admire or even just feeling appreciation that you ate today or have shoes on your feet. If your mind wanders, just bring it gently back to the positive experience.

These three steps, when practised daily for five minutes, can help you to de-stress, feel calmer and more content. Once you've got the hang of the exercise, you can then use it any time you encounter a stressful event; for example, as you start to feel tense in heavy traffic, or if you are overloaded at work or you sense that you are about to face a difficult emotional situation. Just a few HeartMath breaths can help you to stay calm and coherent instead of becoming stressed.

Measuring your coherence

Doing the HeartMath exercise will help you to develop greater 'coherence'.

But how will you know? Childre and McCraty discovered that you could monitor your state of coherence accurately by measuring not your heart rate (the number of beats) but the pattern of activity that exists between heartbeats. This is called your heart rate variability or HRV. (We explored this in Chapter 9.) They developed a simple device, called an Em-Wave monitor, which picks up a signal from your thumb (or you can attach an earphone that clips onto your ear lobe to pick up your HRV to track whether or not you are in this 'coherent' state in which cortisol levels rapidly decline). It's an objective measure of what works, and even the very act of knowing, through biofeedback, helps you calm down. With each heartbeat the device flashes a colour, from red to green, and emits a tone that lets you know when you've gone into a relaxed state. By having that feedback it becomes easier to take a deep breath, or maybe have a more uplifting thought, that takes you out of the high stress/cortisol zone.

There's also an excellent book, *Transforming Stress*, which gives very effective exercises for bringing you into a coherent, de-stressed state. In the UK you can attend workshops called Transforming Stress into Resilience to really hardwire these simple stress-busting techniques or you can consult a practitioner on a one-to-one basis (see Resources).

Practise meditation

Another way to find a more coherent, less stressful state is through meditation. In meditation, you become aware of your thoughts, emotions and physical sensations and, in the process, become detached. There are many ways to approach meditation, although many people find it difficult to stop the 'chattering' in the mind. In some meditative techniques you focus on the breath, in some the heart, and in others the vital-energy centre of the body, known as the tantien in t'ai chi and also called the Kath point by the philosopher Oscar Ichazo. (Ichazo has thoroughly researched methods of generating vital energy, known as chi, and of attaining higher states of consciousness.) Some people also repeat a word or a mantra silently.

Diakath breathing

An example of a technique to induce a more coherent and meditative state is Diakath breathing based on the Kath point. Although not an anatomical point as such, the Kath point is the body's centre of gravity, and by placing one's awareness at this point, rather than in the head as we most often do, it is possible to become aware of the whole body. All the martial arts, in their pure form, are practised with this awareness, which gives a more complete and grounded experience of oneself. You can experience this for yourself by practising the simple breathing exercise shown below.

This breathing exercise (reproduced with the kind permission of Oscar Ichazo) connects the Kath point – the body's centre of equilibrium – with the diaphragm muscle, so that deep breathing becomes natural and effortless. You can practise this exercise at any time, while sitting, standing or lying down, and for as long as you like. You can also practise it unobtrusively during moments of stress. It is an excellent, natural relaxant and energy booster, helping you to feel more connected and in tune.

How to practise Diakath breathing

The diaphragm is a dome-shaped muscle attached to the bottom of the rib cage. The Kath point is located three finger-widths below the belly and 2.5cm (1in) in. If you place your index finger in your belly button your little finger will be in the Kath point. When you put your awareness into this point, it becomes easy to be aware of your entire body.

Ideally, find somewhere quiet first thing in the morning. When breathing, inhale and exhale through your nose. As you inhale, you will expand your lower belly from the Kath point and your diaphragm muscle. This allows the lungs to fill with air from the bottom to the top. As you exhale, the belly and the diaphragm muscle relax, allowing the lungs to empty from top to bottom.

1 Sit comfortably, in a quiet place with your spine straight.

2 Focus your attention on your Kath point.

3 Let your belly expand from the Kath point as you inhale slowly, deeply and effortlessly. Feel your diaphragm being pulled down towards the Kath point as your lungs fill with air from the bottom to the top. On the exhale, relax both your belly and your diaphragm, emptying your lungs from top to bottom.

4 Repeat at your own pace.

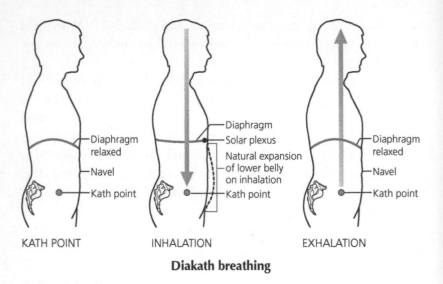

Diakath breathing

When to practise Diakath breathing

- Every morning, sit down in a quiet place before breakfast and practise Diakath breathing for a few minutes.

- Whenever you are stressed throughout the day, check your breathing. Practise Diakath breathing for nine breaths. This is great to do before an important meeting or when something has upset you.

(© 2002 Oscar Ichazo. Diakath breathing is the service mark and Kath the trademark of Oscar Ichazo. Used by permission.)

It's worth finding out what appeals to you

The purpose of such practices is to centre yourself, to take yourself out of small-minded stressful and fearful thoughts, and thus to become of more use to yourself and others. There are, of course, many different ways of doing this, some of which I list in Resources. Exercises such as yoga and t'ai chi are great ways to increase your sense of connection and also to reduce stress. So too is walking the dog, gardening and spending some time in beautiful natural environments.

Case Study: Robert

Robert, aged 66, took up t'ai chi when he retired. Here's how he describes the benefits:

> 'I've never been an athletic person or good at anything physical. T'ai chi, however, I enjoy immensely. I like the feeling of being "in control" of my body. It gives me an aesthetic pleasure. I do it almost every day for 20 minutes. It increases my energy and clears my mind. It gives me a kind of equilibrium that has many benefits, such as helping me to play my violin better and helping me to stay detached when things are bad. I find it very calming when I'm stressed or feeling fraught.'

If stress is a major factor in your life, and affecting your health, you need to make some changes, and learn some ways, such as the above suggestions, for developing a more balanced state of mind as your default. Getting your nutrition right will give you the energy for making these positive changes.

The GL Index of Hundreds of Foods

The most accurate way to gauge whether or not you should eat a food is its glycemic load, which is a calculation based on both the quantity of carbohydrate in a food and the quality of that carbohydrate.

A GL of 10 or less is good, and is shown in **bold**

A GL of 11–14 is OK, shown in normal text

A GL of 15 or more is bad, shown in *italics*

Even this is only a guide, however, because the amount you eat of a food will obviously alter its effect on your blood sugar, and hence your weight. So, while generally I say you can liberally eat the bold foods with low GLs, limit the normal-text foods and avoid the italic foods, what is most important is to limit the *total glycemic load* of your diet. If you want to lose weight and feel great, eat no more than 40 GLs a day. This means roughly 10 for breakfast, 10 for lunch, 10 for dinner and 5 each for your two snacks, mid-morning and mid-afternoon. You can also drink 5 GLs, or have a 5-GL dessert, after the first two weeks or from the start of the diet if you are on insulin, so your total daily intake from food and drink is 45.

If you choose the good, low-GL foods you'll be able to eat more food. If you choose the bad high-GL foods you'll have to eat much less. In the chart below mainly select from the bold foods, then use the right-hand column to work out how much to eat for 5, which is the serving for a snack, or 10, which is a serving for a main meal. If you are not sure what a 'serving' means look at the amounts of grams given for 5 and check the grams on the packet of the food in question. Foods containing no carbohydrate, composed entirely of protein or fat (meat, fish, eggs, cheese, mayonnaise) have, in effect, a GL of 0, and are not included in this chart. Please note that the glycemic index for some foods has not been published. In these instances we have estimated the GL based on the GI for very similar foods. These foods are marked 'E'. As the GLs of more foods are calculated, this table will be updated on www.theholforddiet.com. You can also input a selection of foods into this database and it will calculate the GL of a particular recipe for you.

THE GLYCEMIC LOAD OF COMMON FOODS

Item	Serving size (in g)	GLs per serving	10 GLs	5 GLs	5 GLs
Bakery products					
Muffin – apple, made without sugar	**60**	**9**	**1 muffin**	**½ muffin**	**33g**
Muffin – apple muffin, made with sugar	60	13	1 small muffin	½ small muffin	23g
Crumpet	50	13	1 crumpet	½ crumpet	19g
Muffin – apple, oat, sultana, made from packet mix	50	14	1 small muffin	½ small muffin	18g
Muffin – bran	*57*	*15*	*½ muffin*	*¼ muffin*	*18g*
Muffin – blueberry	*57*	*17*	*½ muffin*	*¼ muffin*	*17g*
Muffin – banana, oat and honey	*50*	*17*	*½ muffin*	*¼ muffin*	*15g*
Muffin – carrot	*57*	*20*	*½ muffin*	*¼ muffin*	*14g*
Banana cake, made without sugar	*80*	*16*	*1 small slice*	*⅓ slice*	*25g*
Croissant	*57*	*17*	*½ croissant*	*¼ croissant*	*17g*
Doughnut	*47*	*17*	*½ doughnut*	*¼ doughnut*	*14g*
Sponge cake, plain	*63*	*17*	*½ slice*	*¼ slice*	*19g*

Breads

Item	Serving size (in g)	GLs per serving	10 GLs	5 GLs	5 GLs
Rye kernel (pumpernickel) bread	30	6	2 slices	1 slice	25g
Sourdough rye	30	6	2 slices	1 slice	25g
Volkenbrot, wholemeal rye bread	30	7	2 slices	1 slice	21g
Rice bread, high-amylose	30	7	2 small slices	1 small slice	21g
Rice bread, low-amylose	30	8	2 thin slices	1 thin slice	19g
Wholemeal rye bread	30	8	2 thin slices	1 thin slice	19g
Wheat tortilla (Mexican)	50	8	1½ tortillas	Less than 1 tortilla	31g
Chapatti, white wheat flour, thin, with green gram	50	8	1½ chapattis	1 chapatti	31g
White, high-fibre	30	9	1 thick slice	1 thin slice	17g
Wholemeal (wholewheat) wheat flour bread	30	9	1 thick slice	1 thin slice	17g
Gluten-free fibre-enriched	30	9	1 thick slice	½ thick slice	17g
Gluten-free multigrain bread	30	10	1 slice	½ slice	15g
Light rye	30	10	1 slice	½ slice	15g
White wheat flour bread	30	10	1 slice	½ slice	15g
Pitta bread, white	30	10	1 pitta	½ slice	15g
Wheat flour flatbread	30	10	1 slice	½ slice	15g
Gluten-free white bread	30	11	1 slice	½ slice	14g

Item	Serving size (in g)	GLs per serving	10 GLs	5 GLs	5 GLs
Corn tortilla	50	12	1 tortilla	½ tortilla	21g
Middle Eastern flatbread	30	15	⅔ slice	⅓ slice	10g
Baguette, white, plain	30	15	1/20 baton	1/40 baton	10g
Bagel, white, frozen	70	25	½ bagel	¼ bagel	14g

Breakfast cereals

Item	Serving size (in g)	GLs per serving	10 GLs	5 GLs	5 GLs
Low-GL Muesli (see page 243) (E)	30	1	As much as you like	As much as you like	100g
Porridge made from rolled oats	30	2	As much as you like	1 very large bowl	75g
Get Up & Go with strawberries and milk (E)	30	5	⅔ pint drink	½ pint drink	190ml
All-Bran™	30	6	2 small servings	1 small serving	25g
Muesli, gluten-free	30	7	2 small servings	1 small serving	21g
Muesli (Alpen)	30	10	1 serving	½ serving	15g
Muesli, Natural	30	10	1 serving	½ serving	15g
Raisin Bran™ (Kellogg's)	30	12	1 small serving	⅓ serving	13g
Weetabix™	30	13	2 biscuits	1 biscuit	12g
Bran Flakes™	30	13	1 small serving	⅓ serving	12g

Item	Serving size (in g)	GLs per serving	10 GLs	5 GLs	5 GLs
Sultana Bran™ (Kellogg's)	30	14	1 small serving	⅔ serving	11g
Special K™ (Kellogg's)	30	14	1 small serving	⅓ serving	11g
Shredded Wheat	30	15	1 biscuit	⅓ serving	10g
Cheerios™	30	15	1 very small serving	⅓ serving	10g
Frosties™, sugar-coated cornflakes (Kellogg's)	30	15	1 very small serving	⅓ serving	10g
Grapenuts™	30	15	1 very small serving	⅓ serving	10g
Golden Wheats™ (Kellogg's)	30	16	1 very small serving	⅓ serving	9g
Puffed Wheat	30	16	1 very small serving	⅓ serving	9g
Honey Smacks™ (Kellogg's)	30	16	1 very small serving	⅓ serving	9g
Cornflakes, Crunchy Nut™ (Kellogg's)	30	17	1 very small serving	⅓ serving	9g
Coco Pops™ (cocoa-flavoured puffed rice)	30	20	½ serving	¼ serving	8g
Rice Krispies™ (Kellogg's)	30	21	½ serving	¼ serving	7g
Cornflakes™ (Kellogg's)	30	21	½ serving	¼ serving	7g

Cereal grains

Semolina	150	6	1 very large serving	small serving	125g
Taco shells, cornmeal-based, baked (Old El Paso)	20	8	2 shells	1 shell	13g
Quinoa	150	8	1½ cups	⅔ cup	94g
Cornmeal	150	9	1 very large serving	1 small serving	83g

Item	Serving size (in g)	GLs per serving	10 GLs	5 GLs	5 GLs
			1 very large serving	1 small serving	
Kamut (E)	**150**	**9**	**1 serving**	**½ serving**	**83g**
Pearl Barley	150	11	1 serving	½ serving	68g
Cracked wheat (bulgur/bourghul)	150	12	1 serving	½ serving	63g
Brown basmati rice	150	13	1 small serving	½ serving	58g
Buckwheat	*150*	*16*	*1 small serving*	*⅓ serving*	*47g*
Rice, brown	*150*	*18*	*1 small serving*	*⅓ serving*	*42g*
Rice, long grain, white, precooked microwaved 2 min.					
(Express Rice, Uncle Ben's)	*150*	*19*	*½ serving*	*¼ serving*	*39g*
Basmati, white, boiled	*150*	*22*	*½ serving*	*¼ serving*	*34g*
Couscous	*150*	*23*	*½ serving*	*¼ serving*	*33g*
Rice, white	*150*	*23*	*½ serving*	*¼ serving*	*33g*
Long grain, boiled	*150*	*23*	*½ serving*	*¼ serving*	*33g*
Millet, porridge	*150*	*25*	*½ serving*	*¼ serving*	*30g*

Crispbreads and crackers

Oatcakes	25	8	4 oatcakes	2 oatcakes	16g
Digestives	**25**	**10**	**1 biscuit**	**½ biscuit**	**13g**
Cream cracker	25	11	2 biscuits	1 biscuit	11g
Rye crispbread	25	11	2 biscuits	1 biscuit	11g

Item	Serving size (in g)	GLs per serving	10 GLs	5 GLs	5 GLs
Water cracker	25	17	2 biscuits	1 biscuit	7g
Puffed rice cakes	*25*	*17*	*2 biscuits*	*1 biscuit*	*7g*

Dairy products and alternatives

Item	Serving size (in g)	GLs per serving	10 GLs	5 GLs	5 GLs
Plain yoghurt (no sugar)	200	3	3 small pots	1½ small pots	333g
Non-fat yoghurt (plain, no sugar)	200	3	3 small pots	1½ small pots	333g
Milk, full-fat	250ml	3	833ml	416ml	416ml
Milk, skim (Canada)	250ml	4	625ml	312ml	312ml
Soya yoghurt (Provamel)	200	7	2 small pots	1 small pot	150g
Soya milk (no sugar)	250ml	7	2 small cups	1 small cup	178ml
Custard, homemade from milk	100ml	7	1 small cup	½ cup	71ml
Ice cream, regular	50ml	8	2 scoops	1 scoop	31ml
Soya milk (sweetened with apple juice concentrate)	250ml	8	2 small cups	1 small cup	156ml
Soya milk, reduced-fat (1.5%), 120mg calcium	250ml	8	2 small cups	1 small cup	156ml
Soya milk (sweetened with sugar)	250ml	9	1½ small cups	⅔ small cup	138ml
Low-fat yoghurt, fruit, sugar, (Ski™)	200	10	1½ small pots	⅔ of small pot	100g
Rice milk, E	250ml	14	1 small cup	½ cup	90ml
Milk, condensed, sweetened (Nestlé)	*50ml*	*17*	*1 tsp*	*½ tsp*	*14ml*

267

Fruit and fruit products

Item	Serving size (in g)	GLs per serving	10 GLs	5 GLs	5 GLs
Blackberries E	120	1	2 large punnets	1 large punnet	600g
Blueberries E	120	1	2 large punnets	1 large punnet	600g
Raspberries E	120	1	2 large punnets	1 large punnet	600g
Strawberries, fresh, raw	120	1	2 large punnets	1 large punnet	600g
Cherries, raw	120	3	2 punnets	1 punnet	200g
Grapefruit, raw	120	3	1 large	1 small	200g
Pear, raw	120	4	2 large pears	1 large pear	150g
Melon/cantaloupe, raw	120	4	1 small melon	½ small melon	150g
Watermelon, raw	120	4	2 big slices	1 big slice	150g
Peaches raw (or canned in natural juice)	120	5	2 peaches	1 peach	120g
Apricots, raw	120	5	8 apricots	4 apricots	120g
Oranges, raw	120	5	2 large	1 large	120g
Plum, raw	120	5	8 plums	4 plums	120g
Apples, raw	120	6	2 small	1 small	100g
Kiwi fruit, raw	120	6	2 kiwis	1 kiwi	100g
Pineapple raw	120	7	2 thin slices	1 thin slice	85g
Grapes, raw	120	8	20 grapes	10 grapes	75g

Item	Serving size (in g)	GLs per serving	10 GLs	5 GLs	5 GLs
Mango, raw	120	8	½ mango	1 slice	75g
Apricots, dried	60	9	6 apricots	3 apricots	33g
Fruit Cocktail, canned (Delmonte)	120	9	Small can	Half a small can	66g
Pawpaw/papaya, raw	120	10	Half a small papaya	1 slice	60g
Prunes, pitted	60	10	6 prunes	3 prunes	30g
Apple, dried	60	10	6 rings	3 rings	30g
Banana, raw	120	12	1 banana	½ banana	50g
Apricots, canned in light syrup	120	12	Less than 1 small can	⅓ small can	50g
Lychees, canned in syrup and drained	120	16	½ 200g can	¼ 200g can	37g
Figs, dried, tenderised, Dessert Maid brand	60	16	2 figs	1 fig	19g
Sultanas	60	25	20	10	12g
Raisins	60	28	20	10	11g
Dates, dried	60	42	2 dates	1 date	7g

Jams and spreads

Item	Serving size (in g)	GLs per serving	10 GLs	5 GLs	5 GLs
Pumpkin seed butter E	16	1	3 large pots	1½ large pots	765g
Peanut butter (no sugar) E	16	1	3 large pots	1½ large pots	765g
Blueberry spread (no sugar) E	30	4	4 tbsp	2 tbsp	21g
Apricot fruit spread, reduced sugar	30	7	8 tsp	4 tsp	21g

Item	Serving size (in g)	GLs per serving	10 GLs	5 GLs	5 GLs
Orange marmalade	30	9	8 tsp	4 tsp	17g
Strawberry jam	30	10	2 tbsp	2 heaped tsp	15g

Legumes and nuts

Item	Serving size (in g)	GLs per serving	10 GLs	5 GLs	5 GLs
Hummus (chickpea dip)	30	1	4 large tubs	4 small tubs	765g
Soya beans	150	1	6 cups	3 cups	750g
Peas, dried, boiled	150	2	3 cups	1½ cups	375g
Pinto beans, boiled in salted water	150	4	2 cups	1 cup	187g
Borlotti beans, boiled, canned	150	4	1½ cans	⅔ can	187g
Lentils	150	5	2 cups	1 cup	150g
Butter beans	150	6	1½ cups	⅔ cup	125g
Split peas, yellow, boiled 20 min.	150	6	1½ cups	⅔ cup	125g
Baked beans, canned	150	7	½ can	¼ can	107g
Kidney beans, canned	150	7	¾ can	⅓ can	107g
Chickpeas (Bengal gram), boiled	150	8	1½ cups	⅔ cup	94g
Chickpeas, canned in brine	150	9	¾ can	⅓ can	83g
Chestnuts, cooked E	150	8	1½ cups	⅔ cup	94g
Flageolet beans, canned in brine E	150	8	¾ can	⅓ can	83g
Haricot/navy beans, canned	150	12	½ can	¼ can	62g
Black-eyed beans, boiled	150	13	1 cup	½ cup	58g

Pasta and noodles*

Item	Serving size (in g)	GLs per serving	10 GLs	5 GLs	5 GLs
Ravioli, durum wheat flour, meat filled, boiled	90	7.5	½ packet	1 small serving	60g
Vermicelli, white, boiled	90	8	1 large serving	½ large serving	56g
Spaghetti, wholemeal, boiled	90	8	1 large serving	½ large serving	56g
Pasta, wholemeal, boiled	90	8	1 large serving	½ a serving	56g
Fettuccine, egg, boiled	90	9	1 serving	½ a serving	50g
Spirali, durum wheat, white, boiled to *al dente* texture	90	9	1 serving	½ serving	47g
Spaghetti, white, boiled	90	9	1 serving	½ serving	47g
Instant noodles	90	9	1 serving	½ serving	47g
Spaghetti durum wheat, boiled 10–15 min,	90	10	1 serving	½ serving	43g
Gluten-free pasta, maize starch, boiled 8 min.	90	11	1 small serving	½ small serving	41g
Macaroni, plain	90	11	1 very small serving	½ very small serving	39g
Rice noodles, dried, boiled	90	11	1 very small serving	½ very small serving	39g
Udon noodles, plain (buckwheat/wheat)	90	15	⅔ serving	⅓ serving	30g
Corn pasta, gluten-free	90	16	1 small serving	½ small serving	28g
Gnocchi	90	16	1 very small serving	½ small serving	27g
Rice pasta, brown, boiled 16 min.	90	17	1 very small serving	½ small serving	26g

Item	Serving size (in g)	GLs per serving	10 GLs	5 GLs	5 GLs
Snack foods (savoury)					
Olives, in brine E	**50**	**1**	**4 cups**	**2 cups**	**270g**
Peanuts	**50**	**1**	**1 large pack**	**1 medium or 2 small packs**	**250g**
Cashew nuts, salted	**50**	**3**	**1½ small packs**	**Less than 1 small pack**	**83g**
Popcorn, salted, no sugar	**20**	**8**	**1 small pack**	**½ small pack**	**12g**
Potato crisps, plain, salted	50	11	1½ small packs	⅔ small pack	23g
Pretzels, oven-baked, traditional wheat flavour	30	16	8 pretzels	4 pretzels	9g
Corn chips, plain, salted	50	17	13 chips	7 chips	15g
Snack foods (sweet)					
Fruitus apple cereal bar E	35	5	2 bars	1 bar	35g
Rebar fruit and veg bar E	50	8	1 bar	½ bar	25g
Muesli bar containing dried fruit	30	13	Less than 1 bar	Less than ½ bar	12g
Chocolate, milk, plain (Mars/Cadburys/Nestlé)	50	14	less than ½ bar	Less than ¼ bar	18g
Apricot fruit bar (dried apricot filling in wholemeal pastry)	50	17	1 bar	½ bar	15g

Item	Serving size (in g)	GLs per serving	10 GLs	5 GLs	5 GLs
Twix ® Cookie Bar, caramel (M&M/Mars, USA)	60	17	*1 stick*	*½ stick*	*18g*
Snickers Bar ®	60	19	*⅔ bar*	*⅓ bar*	*16g*
Polos – peppermint sweets	30	21	*8 polos*	*4 polos*	*7g*
Jellybeans, assorted colours	30	22	*4 jellybeans*	*2 jellybeans*	*7g*
Pop Tarts™, double choc	50	24	*21g*	*10g*	*10g*
Mars Bar ®	60	26	*½ bar*	*¼ bar*	*13g*

SOUPS

Item	Serving size (in g)	GLs per serving	10 GLs	5 GLs	5 GLs
Tomato soup	**250**	**6**	**1 can**	**½ can**	**208g**
Minestrone	**250**	**7**	**1 can**	**½ can**	**179g**
Lentil, canned	**250**	**9**	**⅔ can**	**⅓ can**	**139g**
Split pea, canned	*250*	*16*	*½ can*	*¼ can*	*78g*
Black bean, canned	*250*	*17*	*½ can*	*¼ can*	*74g*
Green pea, canned	*250*	*17*	*½ can*	*¼ can*	*74g*

Sugars

Item	Serving size (in g)	GLs per serving	10 GLs	5 GLs	5 GLs
Xylitol	**20**	**2**	**6 tbsp**	**3 tbsp**	**50g**
Blue agave cactus nectar (liquid sweetener in drinks)	**20**	**2**	**100ml**	**50ml**	**50g**

Item	Serving size (in g)	GLs per serving	10 GLs	5 GLs	5 GLs
Fructose	**20**	**4**	**3 tbsp**	**5 tsp**	**25g**
Sucrose	20	14	3 tsp	1½ tsp	7g
Honey	20	16	2 tsp	1 tsp	6g
Glucose	20	20	2 tsp	1 tsp	5g
Maltose (malt)	20	22	2 tsp	1 tsp	5g

Vegetables

Item	Serving size (in g)	GLs per serving	10 GLs	5 GLs	5 GLs
Tomato E	70	2	5 medium	2½ medium	175g
Broccoli E	100	2	5 handfuls	2½ handfuls	250g
Kale E	75	1	10 handfuls	5 handfuls	375g
Avocado E	190	1	10	5	950g
Onion E	180	2	5 medium	2½ medium	450g
Asparagus E	125	2	5 handfuls	2½ handfuls	315g
Green beans E	75	1	10 handfuls	5 handfuls	375g
Carrots	80	3	2 carrots	1 carrot	133g
Green peas	80	3	5 tbsp	2–3 tbsp	133g
Pumpkin	80	3	3 servings	1½ serving	133g
Beetroot	80	5	4 beets	2 beets	80g
Swede	150	7	½ swede	1 serving	107g

Item	Serving size (in g)	GLs per serving	10 GLs	5 GLs	5 GLs
Banana/plantain, green	120	8	1 small	½ small	75g
Broad beans	80	9	89g	1 tbsp	44g
Sweetcorn	80	9	1 serving	½ serving	44g
Parsnips	80	12	1 small	½ small	33g
Yam	150	13	1 small serving	½ small serving	58g
Boiled potato	150	14	107g	1 small	53g
Microwaved potato	150	14	107g	1 small	53g
Mashed potato	150	15	2 tbsp	1 tbsp	50g
New potato, unpeeled and boiled 20 min.	150	16	4 very small	2 very small	47g
Instant mashed potato	150	17	88g	2 tsp	44g
Sweet potato	150	17	1 small	½ small	44g
Baked potato, white, baked in skin	150	18	83g	⅔ medium	42g
French fries	150	22	68g	4–5	34g
Baked potato, baked without fat	150	26	½ a medium	¼ a medium	29g

TABLE OF GLYCEMIC LOAD (GL) OF COMMON DRINKS

Item	Serving size in ml	GL per serving	10 GLs	5 GLs	5 GLs
DRINKS					
Tomato juice, canned, no added sugar	**250**	**4**	**625ml**	**½ pint**	**315ml**
Yakult ®, fermented milk drink with Lactobacillus casei	**65**	**6**	**108ml**	**⅔ × 65ml bottle**	**30ml**
Smoothie drink, soya, banana	**250**	**7**	**357ml**	**⅔ × 250ml carton**	**175ml**
Smoothie drink, soya, chocolate hazelnut	**250**	**8**	**313ml**	**⅗ × 250ml carton**	**150ml**
Carrot juice, freshly made	**250**	**10**	**250ml**	**⅕ pint or ⅓ cup**	**125ml**
Grapefruit juice, unsweetened	250	11	227ml	⅕ pint or ⅓ cup	115ml
Apple juice, pure, unsweetened	250	12	208ml	⅙ pint or ⅓ cup	105ml
Orange juice	250	13	192ml	⅙ pint or ⅓ cup	95ml
Cordial, orange, reconstituted	250	13	192ml	⅙ pint or ⅓ cup	95ml
Smoothie, raspberry	250	14	179ml	⅖ 250ml carton or ⅓ cup	90ml
Pineapple juice, unsweetened	*250*	*16*	*156ml*	*¼ pint or ½ cup*	*80ml*
Cranberry juice drink, Ocean Spray®	*250*	*16*	*156ml*	*¼ pint or ½ cup*	*80ml*
Coca Cola ®, soft drink/soda	*250*	*16*	*156ml*	*⅕ × 330ml can*	*80ml*
Fanta ®, orange soft drink	*250*	*23*	*109ml*	*⅙ pint or ⅓ cup*	*50ml*
Lucozade ®, original	*250*	*40*	*63*	*⅛ pint or ¼ cup*	*30ml*

Most of the GL values of foods listed here are derived from research published in 2002 by K. Foster-Powell, S.H. Holt and J. C. Brand-Miller in 'International table of glycemic index and glycemic load values: 2002', *American Journal of Clinical Nutrition* Vol. 76(1) (2002), pp. 5–56 or from the University of Sydney online database at http://www.glycemicindex.com/ (database pages created by A/Prof. Gareth Denyer and Scott Dickirson using data collected by Professor Jennie Brand-Miller & SUGIRS). Last modified: 13 December 2005.

Notes

Serving sizes:

* All pasta serving sizes are for cooked food. For the equivalent of dry weight, halve the amount – so, if you're cooking spaghetti and the serving size is 120g, that means you put 60g in the pan.

Personalising Your GL Intake

Even though I've recommended you eat between 40 and 45 GLs a day in total in order to lose weight, the truth is that your ideal daily GL is whatever keeps your blood sugar level in check. Also, it will vary according to your weight and the amount of exercise you do. The chart below shows you your ideal daily GL to lose weight and stabilise your blood sugar, according to your weight and frequency of exercise.

Your ideal daily GL intake to lose weight according to your height and activity level

		Average exercise per day (mins)						
		0	**15**	**30**	**45**	**60**	**90**	**120**
	5 ft (1.52m)	35	35	40	45	45	50	55
	5 ft 3 (1.60m)	40	40	40	45	50	55	60
	5 ft 6 (1.67m)	40	40	40	45	50	55	60
Height	5 ft 9 (1.75m)	40	40	45	50	55	60	65
	6 ft (1.83m)	45	45	50	55	60	65	70
	6 ft 3 (1.91m)	50	50	55	60	65	70	75
	6 ft 6 (1.98m)	55	55	60	65	70	75	80

References

Introduction

1. Coronary heart disease statistics in England, February 2011, British Heart Foundation – see www.bhf.org.uk
2. H. Tunstall-Pedoe, et al., 'Contribution of trends in survival and coronary-event rates to changes in coronary heart disease mortality: 10-year results from 37 WHO MONICA project populations. Monitoring trends and determinants in cardiovascular disease', *Lancet*, 1999;353:1517–57

Part 1

1. A. Sachdeva, et al., 'Lipid levels in patients hospitalized with coronary artery disease: An analysis of 136,905 hospitalizations in Get With The Guidelines'. *American Heart Journal*, 2009 Jan;157(1):111–17
2. W. De Ruijter, et al., 'Use of Framingham risk score and new biomarkers to predict cardiovascular mortality in older people: population based observational cohort study', *British Medical Journal*, 2009 Jan 8;338:a3083
3. S. Yusuf, et al., 'Effect of potentially modifiable risk factors associated with myocardial infarction in 52 countries (the INTERHEART study): Case-control study', *Lancet*, 2004 Sep;364(9438):937–52
4. M. McQueen, et al., 'Lipids, lipoproteins, and apolipoproteins as risk markers of myocardial infarction in 52 countries (the INTERHEART study): A case-control study', *Lancet*, 2008 Jul 19;372(9634):224–33
5. T. Forsén, et al., 'Mother's weight in pregnancy and coronary heart disease in a cohort of Finnish men: Follow-up study,' *British Medical Journal*, 1997;l315:837–40
6. M. Cannon, et al., 'The effect of combined micronutrient supplementation on blood pressure' (1990), paper held at ION Library, available from ION, Richmond, Surrey
7. M. Colgan, Institute of Nutritional Science, unpublished material held in ION library
8. E. Cheraskin, et al., 'The biologic parabola: A look at serum cholesterol', *Journal of the American Medical Association*, 1982;247(3):302
9. E.J. Parks, et al., 'Dietary sugars stimulate fatty acid synthesis in adults', *Journal of Nutrition*, 2008 Jun;138(6):1039–46
10. E.S. Ford, et al., 'Hypertriglyceridemia and its pharmacologic treatment among US adults', *Archives of Internal Medicine*, 2009;169(6):572–8

11. S. Mottillo, K.B. Filion, et al.,'The metabolic syndrome and cardiovascular risk: A systematic review and meta-analysis', *Journal of the American College of Cardiology*, 2010 Sep;56(14):1113–32

12. Reported at the International Congress of Nutrition in Kyoto, Japan 1975 by Dr R. Alfin-Slater

13. http://www.surrey.ac.uk/mediacentre/press/2009/2840_twoegg_diet_cracks_cholesterol_issue.htm

14. R.H. Knopp, B.M. Retzlaff, et al., 'A double-blind, randomized, controlled trial of the effects of two eggs per day in moderately hypercholesterolemic and combined hyperlipidemic subjects taught the NCEP step I diet', *Journal of the American College of Nutrition*, 1997 Dec;16(6):551–61

15. De Oliviera e Silva, et al., 'Effects of shrimp consumption on plasma lipoproteins', *American Journal of Clinical Nutrition*, 1996;64(5):712–17

16. Report of the Advisory Panel of the Committee on Medical Aspects of Food Policy on Diet in Relation to Cardiovascular and Cerebrovascular Disease. *Diet and Coronary Heart Disease*, London, 1974.

17. A. Qureshi, F.K. Suri, et al., 'Regular egg consumption does not increase the risk of stroke and cardiovascular diseases', *Medical Science Monitor*, 2006;13(1):CR1–8; also L. Djoussél and J. Michael Gaziano, 'Egg consumption and cardiovascular disease and mortality: The Physicians' Health Study', *American Journal of Clinical Nutrition*, 2008 Apr;87(4): 964–969; also D.K. Houston, et al., 'Dietary fat and cholesterol and risk of cardiovascular disease in older adults: The Health ABC Study', *Nutrition, Metabolism and Cardiovascular Disease*, 2011 Jun;21(6): 430–7; also C. Scrafford, et al., 'Egg consumption and CHD and stroke mortality: A prospective study of US adults', *Public Health Nutrition*, 2011 Feb;14(2):261–70

18. W. Willetts, 'The great fat debate: Total fat and health', *Journal of the American Medical Association*, May 2011;111(5):660–2

19. WHO Geneva, 'Interim Summary of Conclusions and Dietary Recommendations on Total Fat and Fatty Acids' from the Joint FAO/WHO Expert Consultation on Fats and Fatty Acids in Human Nutrition, 2008 Nov

20. P.W. Siri-Tarino, et al., 'Saturated fat, carbohydrate, and cardiovascular disease', *American Journal of Clinical Nutrition*, 2010 Mar;91(3):502–9

21. A. Sachdeva, et al., 'Lipid levels in patients hospitalized with coronary artery disease: An analysis of 136,905 hospitalizations in Get With The Guidelines' *American Heart Journal*, 2009 Jan;157(1):111–117.e2

22. W. de Ruijter, et al., 'Use of Framingham risk score and new biomarkers to predict cardiovascular mortality in older people: Population based observational cohort study', *British Medical Journal*, 2009 Jan;338:a3083

23. M.K. Jain and P. M. Ridke, 'Anti-inflammatory effects of statins: Clinical evidence and basic mechanisms', *Nature Reviews Drug Discovery*, 2005 Dec;4:977–87

24. For a detailed discussion of the complex role of cholesterol in the body and a critical analysis of the big trials usually used to support statin use, see a long and authoritative article by biochemists and nutrition authors Sally Fallon and Mary Enig at: http://westonaprice.org/cardiovascular-disease/dangers-of-statin-drugs.html

25. See http://www.fao.org/docrep/V4700E/V4700E0i.htm

26. E.C. Suarez, 'Relations of trait depression and anxiety to low lipid and lipoprotein concentrations in healthy young adult women', *Psychosomatic Medicine*,1999;61(3):273–9

27. T. Partonen, et al., 'Association of low serum total cholesterol with major depression and suicide', *British Journal of Psychiatry*, 1999;175:259–62

28. L. Buydens-Branchey, M. Branchey, et al., 'Low HDL cholesterol, aggression and altered central serotonergic activity', *Psychiatry Research,* 2000 Mar;93(2):93–102

29. K. Carroll, et al., 'Stroke incidence and risk factors in a population based cohort study', *Health Statistics Quarterly*, 2001;12:18–26

30. C. Wolfe, 'The Burden of Stroke' in C. Wolfe, T. Rudd, and R. Beech (eds), *Stroke Services and Research* (1996), The Stroke Association

31. *Stroke Statistics,* British Heart Foundation and The Stroke Association, 2009

32. *Coronary Heart Disease Statistics*, British Heart Foundation, 2005

33. M.R. Law, et al., 'Quantifying effect of statins on low density lipoprotein cholesterol, ischaemic heart disease, and stroke: Systematic review and meta-analysis', *British Medical Journal*, 2003 Jun;326(7404):1423

34. K. Johnson, et al., 'Traditional clinical risk assessment tools do not accurately predict coronary atherosclerotic plaque burden: A CT angiography study', *American Journal of Roentgenology,* 2009 Jan;192(1): 235–43

35. *Metro newspaper*, front page 14 March 2006

36. P. Thavendriranathan, et al., 'Primary Prevention of Cardiovascular Diseases With Statin Therapy ', *Archives of Internal Medicine*, 2006 Nov;166:2307–2313, also see reference 43 below.

37. J. Abramson and J. Wright. 'Are lipid-lowering guidelines evidence-based?', *Lancet* 2007;369:168–9

38. K. Kausik, et al., 'Statins and all-cause mortality in high-risk primary prevention: A meta-analysis of 11 randomized controlled trials involving 65 229 participants', *Archives of Internal Medicine*, 2010;170(12):1024–31

39. I. Gissi-HF, et al., 'Effect of n-3 polyunsaturated fatty acids in patients with chronic heart failure (theGISSI-HF trial): A randomised, double-blind, placebo-controlled trial', *Lancet,* 2008;372(9645):1223–30; also GISSI-HF investigators, 'Effect of rosuvastatin in patients with chronic heart failure (the GISSI-HF trial): A randomized, double-blind, placebo-controlled trial', *Lancet,* 2008. Available at: http://www.thelancet.com http://www.theheart.org/viewDocument.do?document=http%3A%2F%2Fwww.thelancet.com

40. I. Ford, et al., 'Long-term follow-up of the West of Scotland coronary prevention study', *New England Journal of Medicine*, 2007 Oct;357(15):1477–86

41. See P. Langsjoen,'Introduction to coenzyme Q10', at http://faculty. washington.edu/~ely/coenzq10.html

42. P.H. Langsjoen, 'Statin-induced cardiomyopathy', *Redflagsweekly.com*, 8 July 2002

43. F. Taylor, et al., 'Statins for the primary prevention of cardiovascular disease', *Cochrane Database Systematic Review*, 2011;1(CD004816)

44. D. Graveline, *Lipitor: Thief of memory, statin drugs and the misguided war on cholesterol*, Infinity Publishing, 2004

45. U. Ravnskov, et al., 'Analysis and comment controversy: Should we lower cholesterol as much as possible?', *British Medical Journal*, 2006;332:1330–2

46. B. Golomb, et al, 'Physician response to patient reports of adverse drug effects: Implications for patient-targeted adverse effect surveillance', *Drug Safety*, 2007;30(8)669–75

47. A.A. Alsheikh-Ali, et al., 'Effect of the magnitude of lipid lowering on risk of elevated liver enzymes, rhabdomyolysis, and cancer: Insights from large randomized statin trials', *Journal of the American College of Cardiology*, 2007;50409–18

48. D. Mangin, et al., 'Preventive health care in elderly people needs rethinking', *British Medical Journal*, 2007;335:285–7

49. M.A. Silver, et al., 'Effect of atorvastatin on left ventricular diastolic function and ability of coenzyme Q10 to reverse that dysfunction', *American Journal of Cardiology*, 2004 Nov;94(10):1306–10

50. P.H. Langsjoen, et al., 'Treatment of statin adverse effects with supplemental Coenzyme Q10 and statin drug discontinuation', *Biofactors*, 2005; 25(1–4):147–52

51. NIH News: NIH stops clinical trial on combination cholesterol treatment Embargoed for release 26 May 2011, http//public.nhibi.nih.gov/newsroom/home

52. R.H. Grimm Jr, 'Hypertension management in the Multiple Risk Factor Intervention Trial (MRFIT): Six-year intervention results for men in special intervention and usual care groups', *Archives of Internal Medicine*, 1985;145(7), 1191–9

53. C.D. Furberg, ALLHAT Officers and Coordinators for the ALLHAT Collaborative Research Group, 'Major outcomes in moderately hypercholesterolemic, hypertensive patients randomized to pravastatin vs usual care: The Antihypertensive and Lipid-Lowering Treatment to Prevent Heart Attack Trial (ALLHAT-LLT)', *Journal of the American Medical Association*, 2002;288(23):2998–3007

54. Multiple Risk Factor Intervention Trial Research Group, 'Baseline rest electrocardiographic abnormalities, antihypertensive treatment, and mortality in the Multiple Risk Factor Intervention Trial,' *American Journal of Cardiology*, 1985 Jan;1;55(1):1–15; also J.A. Cutler, et al., 'Coronary

heart disease and all-causes mortality in the Multiple Risk Factor Intervention Trial: Subgroup findings and comparisons with other trials', *American Journal of Preventive Medicine*, 1985 May;14(3):293–311; also R.H. Grimm, et al., 'Hypertension management in the Multiple Risk Factor Intervention Trial (MRFIT): Six-year intervention results for men in special intervention and usual care groups', *Archives of Internal Medicine*, 1985 Jul;145(7):1191–9; also, no authors listed, 'Mortality after 10 1/2 years for hypertensive participants in the Multiple Risk Factor Intervention Trial', *Circulation*, 1990 Nov;82(5):1616–28.

55. R. Burton, 'Withdrawing antihypertensive treatment', *British Medical Journal*, 1991;303:324–5

56. S. Bangalore, S. Sawhney, et al., 'Relation of beta-blocker induced heart rate lowering and cardioprotection in hypertension', *Journal of the American College of Cardiology*, 2008;52:1482–89

57. C.D. Furberg, et al., 'Nifedipine: Dose-related increase in mortality in patients with coronary heart disease', *Circulation*, 1995;92(5):1326–33

58. *Guardian*, 'Medical error may have caused Sharon's stroke' 21 April 2006

59. Fowkes, et al., 'Aspirin for Prevention of Cardiovascular events in a General Population Screened for a Low Ankle Brachial Index', *Journal of the American Medical Association*, 2010 Mar;303(9): 841–8

60. C. Baigent, L. Blackwell, et al., Antithrombotic Trialists' (ATT) Collaboration, 'Aspirin in the primary and secondary prevention of vascular disease: Collaborative meta-analysis of individual participant data from randomised trials', *Lancet*, 2009 May;373(9678):1849–60

61. H. Barnett, P. Burrill, et al., 'Don't use aspirin for primary prevention of cardiovascular disease', *British Medical Journal*, 2010;340:c1805

62. C. Shing Kwok and Y.K. Loke, 'Critical Overview on the Benefits and Harms of Aspirin', *Pharmaceuticals*, 2010;3:1491–1506

63. J.S. Berger, A. Lala, et.al., 'Aspirin for the prevention of cardiovascular events in patients without clinical cardiovascular disease: A meta-analysis of randomized trials', *American Heart Journal*, 2011 Jul;162(1):115–22

64. L.A. Rodríguez, L. Cea-Soriano, et al., 'Discontinuation of low dose aspirin and risk of myocardial infarction: case-control study in UK primary care', *British Medical Journal*, 2011 Jul;343 d4094.

65. British National Formulary (published by British Medical Association and the Royal Pharmaceutical Society of Great Britain)

Part 2

1. H. Sinclair, *Drugs Affecting Lipid Metabolism*, (1980) ARIPS Press

2. Hirai, et al., 'Eicosapentanoeic acid and platelet function in Tapanese, *Lancet*, 1980 Nov;316(8204):1132–3

3. H. Kato, et al., 'Epidemiologic studies of coronary heart disease and stroke in Japanese men living in Japan, Hawaii and California', *American Journal of Epidemiology*, 1973;97(6/73):372–85

4.   C. Albert et al. 'Dietary ALA risk of coronary heart disease' *Circulation*. 2005;112:3232–3238

5.   D. Kromhout et al., 'n-3 fatty acids and cardiovascular events', *New England Journal of Medicine* 2010;363:201526

6.   T. Sanders and K. Younger, 'The effect of dietary supplements of Ω3 polyunsaturated fatty acids on the fatty acid composition of platelets and plasma choline phosphoglycerides', *British Journal of Nutrition*, 1981;45:613

7.   A. Lewis, et al., 'Treatment of hypertriglyceridemia with omega-3 fatty acids: A systemic review', *Journal of the American Academy of Nurse Practitioners*, 2004 Sept;16(9):384–95

8.   Briefing paper on N-3 fatty acids and health, British Nutrition Foundation, July 1999

9.   R. Saynor and D. Verel, 'Effect of a marine oil high in eicosapentaenoic acid on blood lipids and coagulation', *IRCS Medical Science*, 1980;8:378–379; see also R. Saynor and D. Verel, et al., *Haematology*, 1981;46(91):65, and personal communication

10. Gissi-Hf Investigators, 'Effect of n-3 polyunsaturated fatty acids in patients with chronic heart failure (the GISSI-HF trial): A randomised, double-blind, placebo-controlled trial', *Lancet*, 2008 Aug;372(9645):1223–30

11. M. Yokoyama, Origasa, 'Effects of eicosapentaenoic acid on major coronary events in hypercholesterolaemic patients (JELIS): a randomised open-label, blinded endpoint analysis', *Lancet*, 2007 Mar;369(9567):1090–8

12. Gruppo Italiano per lo Studio della Sopravvivenza nell'Infarto Mio-cardico, 'Dietary supplementation with n-3 polyunsaturated fatty acids and vitamin E after myocardial infarction: Results of the GISSI-Prevenzione trial', *Lancet*, 1999;354:447–55

13. J.N. Din, et al., 'Omega-3 fatty acids and cardiovascular disease-fishing for a natural treatment', *British Medical Journal*, 2004 Jan;328:30

14. L. Hooper, et al., 'Risks and benefits of omega-3 fats for mortality, cardiovascular disease, and cancer: Systematic review', *British Medical Journal*, 2006 Mar;332:752

15. M. S. Buckley, et al., 'Fish oil interaction with warfarin', *Ann Pharmacotherapy*, 2004;38(1): 50–52

16. D.S. Grimes, E. Hindle, et al., 'Sunlight, cholesterol and coronary heart disease', *Quarterly Journal of Medicine*, 996;89:579–89

17. J.H. Lee, et al., 'Vitamin D deficiency: An important, common, and easily treatable cardiovascular risk factor?', *Journal of the American College of Cardiology*, 2008;52(24):1949–56

18. J.H. Lee, et al., 'Prevalence of vitamin D deficiency in patients with acute myocardial infarction', *American Journal of Cardiology*, 2011;107(11):1636–8

19. M. Leu, E. Giovannucci, 'Vitamin D: Epidemiology of cardiovascular risks and events', *Best Practice & Research. Clinical Endocrinology & Metabolism*, 2011 Aug;25(4):633–46; see also: J.C. Temmerman, 'Vitamin D and cardiovascular disease', *Journal of the American College of Nutrition*, 2011 Jun;30(3):167–70.

20. S. Maiya, et al., 'Hypocalcaemia and vitamin D deficiency: An important, but preventable, cause of life-threatening infant heart failure', *Heart* 2008;94(5):581–4

21. I. Al Mheid, et al., 'Vitamin D status is associated with arterial stiffness and vascular dysfunction in healthy humans', *Journal of the American College of Cardiology*, 2011;58(2):186–92

22. T.L. Halton, et al., 'Low-carbohydrate-diet score and the risk of coronary heart disease in women', *New England Journal of Medicine*, 2006; 355: 1991–2002

23. S. Liu, et al., 'A prospective study of dietary glycemic load, carbohydrate intake and risk of coronary heart disease in US women', *American Journal of Clinical Nutrition*, 2000;6:1455–61

24. M. Pereira, et al., 'Low-glycemic load diet and resting energy expenditure' *Journal of the American Medical Association*, 2004, 292:2482–90

25. S.A. LaHaye, et al. 'Comparison between a low glycemic load diet and a Canada Food Guide diet in cardiac rehabilitation patients in Ontario', *Canadian Journal of Cardiology*, 2005;21(6):489–94

26. D. Pawlak, et al., 'Effects of dietary glycaemic index on adiposity, glucose homoeostasis, and plasma lipids in animals', *Lancet*, 2004;364(9436):778–85

27. Y. Ma, et al., 'Association between carbohydrate intake and serum lipids', *Journal of the American College of Nutrition*, 2006;25(2):155–163

28. R. Estruch, M.A., Rodriguez-Gonzalez, et al., 'Effects of a Mediterranean-style diet on cardiovascular risk factors: A randomized trial', *Annals of Internal Medicine*, 2006;145(1):1–11

29. S.W. Rizkalla, L. Taghrid, et al., 'Effects of dietary glycaemic index on adiposity, glucose homoeostasis, and plasma lipids in animals', *Diabetes Care*, 2004 Aug;27(8):1866–72

30. S. Sieri, V. Krogh, et al., 'Dietary glycemic load and index and risk of coronary heart disease in a large Italian cohort: The EPICOR study', *Archives of Internal Medicine*, 2010 Apr;170(7):640–7

31. K.N. Burger, et al., 'Dietary glycemic load and glycemic index and risk of coronary heart disease and stroke in Dutch men and women: The EPIC-MORGEN Study', *Public Library of Science One*, 2011;6(10):e25955.

32. G.D. Brinckworth, et al., 'Long-term effects of a very low-carbohydrate diet and a low-fat diet on mood and cognitive function', *Archives of Internal Medicine*, 2009;169(20):1873–80

33. D. Thomas, et al., 'Low glycaemic index or low glycaemic load diets for overweight and obese', *Cochrane Database Systematic Reviews*, 2007;3:CD005105

34. Y.Huang, et al., 'Glycated hemoglobin A1c, fasting plasma glucose, and two-hour postchallenge plasma glucose levels in relation to carotid intima-media thickness in Chinese with normal glucose tolerance', *Journal of Clinical Endocrinology Metabolysm*, 2011 Sep;96(9):E1461–5

35. B. Zethelius, et al., 'A new model for 5-year risk of cardiovascular disease in type 2 diabetes, from the Swedish National Diabetes Register (NDR)', *Diabetes Research Clinical Practice*, 2011 Aug;93(2):276–84

36. E. Selvin, et al., 'Glycated hemoglobin, diabetes, and cardiovascular risk in nondiabetic adults', *New England Journal of Medicine*, 2010 Mar;362(9):800–11

37. C.L. Rohlfing, et al., 'Use of GHb (HbAlc) in screening for undiagnosed diabetes in the U.S. population', *Diabetes Care*, 2000;23:187–97

38. N. Sarwar, et al., 'Markers of dysglycaemia and risk of coronary heart disease in people without diabetes: Reykjavik prospective study and systematic review', *Public Library of Science and Medicine*, 2010 May;7(5):e1000278

39. R. Nishimura, et al., 'Relationship between haemoglobin Alc and cardiovascular disease in mild-to-moderate hypercholesterolemic Japanese individuals: Subanalysis of a large-scale randomized controlled trial', *Cardiovascular Diabetology*, 2011 Jun;10–58

40. I. Gigleux, et al., 'Comparison of a dietary portfolio diet of cholesterol-lowering foods and a statin on LDL particle size phenotype in hypercholesterolaemic participants', *British Journal of Nutrition*, 2007 Dec;98(6):1229–36

41. See http://www.telegraph.co.uk/news/worldnews/1470831/Stress-does-increase-risk-of-heart-attack.html Telegraph.co.uk/news/main.jhtml?xml=/news/2004/09/02/wstres02.xml&sSheet=/portal/2004/2004/09/02/ixportal.html

42. A. Rosengren, et al., 'Association of psychosocial risk factors with risk of acute myocardial infarction in 11119 cases and 13648 controls from 52 countries (the INTERHEART study): Case-control study', *Lancet*, 2004 Sep 11–17;364(9438):953–62

43. C. Aboa-Eboule, et al., 'Job strain and risk of acute recurrent coronary heart disease events', *Journal of the American Medical Association*, 2007;298(14):1652–60

44. N. Vogelzangs, et al., 'Urinary cortisol and six-year risk of all-cause and cardiovascular mortality', *Journal of Clinical Endocrinology and Metabolism*, 2010;95(11):4959–64

45. 100% Health Survey, Holford & Associates, 2010 – see http://www.patrickholford.com/index.php/shop/bookdetail/614/

46. H. Eysenck. 'Scientific evidence demonstrating the link between mental and emotional attitudes, physiological health and long-term well-being', *British Journal of Medical Psychology*, 1988;61(Pt 1)

47. M.A. Mittleman, et al., 'Triggering of acute myocardial infarction onset by episodes of anger', *Circulation*,1995;92(7):1720–5

48. L.D. Kubzansky, et al., 'Is worrying bad for your heart? A prospective study of worry and coronary heart disease in the Normative Aging Study', *Circulation*, 1997 Feb 18;95(4):818–24

49. T. Allison, et al., 'Medical and economic costs of psychologic distress in patients with coronary artery disease', *Mayo Clinic Proceedings*, 1995;70(8)

50. R. McCraty, et al., 'The impact of a new emotional self-management program on stress, emotions, heart-rate variability, dhea and cortisol, integrative' *Physiological and Behavioural Science*, 1998;33(2):151–70

51. R. McCraty, et al., 'Impact of workplace stress reduction program on blood pressure and emotional health in hypertensive employees', *Journal of Alternative and Complementary Medicine*, 2003;9(3):355–69

52. Study carried at the Pacemaker Clinic for Kaiser Hospitals in Orange County, California and featured in the HeartMath Interventions manual, *HeartMath LLC*, 2008:46

53. Frederic Luskin, et al., 'A controlled pilot study of stress management training of elderly patients with congestive heart failure' *Preventive Cardiology*, 2002;5(4):168–72

54. R.H. Schneider, et al.,' Stress reduction in the secondary prevention of cardiovascular disease', *Archives of Internal Medicine*, 2011

55. A.G. Bostom, et al., 'The Framingham Study', *Annals of Internal Medicine*, 1999;131: 352–5 and *International Journal of Clinical Practice*, 2001;55(4): 262–8

56. D. Wald, et al., 'Homocysteine and cardiovascular disease: Evidence on causality from a meta-analysis', *British Medical Journal*, 2002 Nov;325:1202

57. W. De Ruijter, et al., 'Use of Framingham risk score and new biomarkers to predict cardiovascular mortality in older people: Population based observational cohort study', *British Medical Journal*, 2009 Jan 8;338:a3083

58. V. Veeranna, S.K. Zalawadiya, et al., 'Homocysteine and reclassification of cardiovascular disease risk', *Journal of the American College of Cardiology*, 2011 Aug;58(10):1025–33

59. K. Karolczak and B. Olas, 'Mechanism of action of homocysteine and its thiolactone in hemostasis system', *Physiological Research*, 2009;58:623–33

60. S.R. Lentz, 'Mechanisms of homocysteine-induced atherothrombosis', *Journal of Thrombosis and Haemostasis*, 3: 1646–54

61. B. Mutus, et al., 'Homocysteine-induced inhibition of nitric oxide production in platelets: A study on healthy and diabetic subjects', *Diabetologia*, 2001;44,(8): 979–82

62. J. Perla-Kajan, et al., 'Mechanisms of homocysteine toxicity in humans', *Amino Acids*, 2007;32:561–72

63. D. Handy, et al., 'Epigenetic modifications: Basic mechanisms and role in cardiovascular disease', *Circulation*, 2011;123:2145–56

64. N. Li, et al., 'Effects of homocysteine on intracellular nitric oxide and superoxide levels in the renal arterial endothelium', *American Journal of Physiology, Heart and Circulatory Physiology*, 2002;283:1237–43

65. *Newsweek*, 11 August 1997

66. J. Selhub, et al., 'Association between plasma homocysteine concentrations and extracranial carotid artery stenosis', *New England Journal of Medicine* 1995;332(5):286–291

67. I. Graham, et al., 'Plasma homocysteine as a risk factor for vascular disease', *Journal of the American Medical Association*, 1997;277(22):1775–81

68. L.L. Humphrey, R. Fu, et al., 'Homocysteine level and coronary heart disease incidence: A systematic review and meta-analysis' *Mayo Clinic Proceedings*, 2008 Nov;83(11):1203–12

69. A.J. Martí-Carvajal, I. Solà, et al., 'Homocysteine lowering interventions for preventing cardiovascular events' *Cochrane Database of Systematic Reviews* 2009;4: CD006612

70. X. Wang, et al., 'Efficacy of folic acid supplementation in stroke prevention: A meta-analysis', *Lancet*, 2007;369(9576):1876–81

71. D.S. Wald, et al., 'Reconciling the evidence on serum homocysteine and ischaemic heart disease: A meta-analysis', *Public Library of Science ONE*, 2011;6(2):e16473

72. B. Debreceni, L. Debreceni, 'Why do homocysteine-lowering B vitamin and antioxidant E vitamin supplementations appear to be ineffective in the prevention of cardiovascular diseases?', *Cardiovasularc Therapeutics* 2011 Apr [Epub ahead of print]. See also G. Hankey, et al., 'Antiplatelet Therapy and the effects of B vitamins in patients with previous stroke or transient ischaemic attack: a post-hoc subanalysis of VITATOPS, a randomised, placebo-controlled trial', *Lancet*, 2012 May, DOI:10.1016/51474-4422(12)70091-1, published online

73. B.G. Nordestgaard, et al., 'Lipoprotein(a) as a cardiovascular risk factor: current status', *European Heart Journal*. 2010 Dec;31(23):2844–53

74. E. Balogh, et al., 'Interaction between homocysteine and lipoprotein(a) increases the prevalence of coronary artery disease/myocardial infarction in women: A case-control study', *Thrombosis Research*, 2012 Feb;129(2):133–8

75. J. Danesh, R. Collins, et al., 'Lipoprotein(a) and coronary heart disease: Meta-analysis of prospective studies', *Circulation*, 2000;102:1082–1085

76. B.G. Nordestgaard, M.J. Chapman, et al., 'Lipoprotein(a) as a cardiovascular risk factor: Current status', *European Journal of Heart Failure*, 2010 Dec;31(23):2844–53

77. M. Rath, L. Pauling, 'A unified theory of human cardiovascular disease leading the way to the abolition of this disease as a cause of human mortality', *Journal of Orthomolecular Medicine*, 1992;7(1):5–12

78. M. Rath and L. Pauling, 'Hypothesis: Lipoprotein (a) is a surrogate for ascorbate', *Proceedings of the National Academy of Sciences of the USA*, 1990 Aug;87:6204–7

79. R. Lawn, 'Lipoprotein(a) in heart disease', *Scientific American*, 1992 Jun;26–32

80. G.H. Tofler, J.J. Stec, et al., 'The effect of vitamin C supplementation on coagulability and lipid levels in healthy male subjects', *Thrombosis Research*, 2000 Oct;100(1):35–41

81. M. Afkhami-Ardekani, A. Shojaoddiny-Ardekani, 'Effect of vitamin C on blood glucose, serum lipids & serum insulin in type 2 diabetes patients', *Indian Journal of Medical Research*, 2007 Nov;126(5):471–4

82. H. Abdollahzad, S. Eghtesadi, et al., 'Effect of vitamin C supplementation on oxidative stress and lipid profiles in hemodialysis patients', *International Journal for Vitamin and Nutrition Research*, 2009 Sep;79(5–6):281–7

83. S.P. Azen, D. Qian, 'Effect of supplementary antioxidant vitamin intake on carotid arterial wall intima-media thickness in a controlled clinical trial of cholesterol lowering', *Circulation*, 1996 Nov;94(10):2369–72; see also: I.

Ellingsen, I. Seljeflot, 'Vitamin C consumption is associated with less progression in carotid intima media thickness in elderly men: A 3-year intervention study', *Nutrition, Metabolism, and Cardiovascular Diseases*, 2009 Jan;19(1):8–14

84.   E. Porkkala-Sarataho, J.T. Salonen, et al., 'Long-term effects of vitamin E, vitamin C, and combined supplementation on urinary 7-hydro-8-oxo-2'-deoxyguanosine, serum cholesterol oxidation products, and oxidation resistance of lipids in nondepleted men', *Arteriosclerosis, Thrombosis, and Vascular Biology*, 2000;20:2087–93

85.   Y. Kubota, 'Dietary intakes of antioxidant vitamins and mortality from cardiovascular disease: The Japan Collaborative Cohort Study (JACC) study', *Stroke*, 2011 Jun;42(6):1665–72

86.   R.M. Salonen, K. Nyyssönen, et al., 'Six-year effect of combined vitamin C and E supplementation on atherosclerotic progression: The Antioxidant Supplementation in Atherosclerosis Prevention (ASAP) Study', *Circulation*, 2003 Feb;107(7):947–53

87.   S.P. Juraschek et al., 'Effects of vitamin C supplementation on blood pressure: a meta-analysis of randomised controlled trials', *American Journal of Clinical Nutrition* 2012 May;95(5):1079–88

88.   A.G. Bostom, A.L. Hume, 'The effect of high-dose ascorbate supplementation on plasma lipoprotein(a) levels in patients with premature coronary heart disease', *Pharmacotherapy*, 1995 Jul-Aug;15(4):458–64

89.   http://www.orthomolecular.org/library/jom/1993/pdf/1993-v08n03-p137.pdf

90.   D. Holmes, 'An answer to angina,' *Holistic Health*, 1995;49:20–3

91.   E. Mah, M.D. Matos, et al., 'Vitamin C status is related to proinflammatory responses and impaired vascular endothelial function in healthy, college-aged lean and obese men' *Journal of the American Dietetic Association*, 2011 May;111(5):737–43

92.   V. Ivanov et al., 'Anti-atherogenic effects of a mixture of ascorbic acid, lysine, proline, arginine, cysteine, and green tea phenolics in human smooth muscle cells', *Journal of Cardiovascular Pharmacology*, 2007 Mar;49(3):140–5

93.   L. Carlson et al., 'Pronounced lowering of Lp(a) in hyperlipidaemic subjects treated with niacin', *Journal of Internal Medicine*, 1989 Oct;226(4):271–6

94.   I. Gouni-Berthold, HK Berthold, 'Lipoprotein(a): Current perspectives', *Current Vascular Pharmacology*, 2011 Nov;9(6):682–92

95.   M.D. Ashen and R.S. Blumentahl, 'Clinical practice: Low HDL cholesterol levels', *New England Journal of Medicine*, 2005;353(12):1252–60

96.   M.J. Chapman, et al., 'Niacin and fibrates in atherogenic dyslipidemia: Pharmacotherapy to reduce cardiovascular risk', *Pharmacology & Therapeutics*, 2010;126(3):314–45

97.   P.L. Canner, K.G. Berge, et al., 'Fifteen year mortality in Coronary Drug Project patients: Long-term benefit with niacin', *Journal of the American College of Cardiology*, 1986;8:1245–55

98.   M. John Chapman, P. Giral, et al., 'Niacin and fibrates in atherogenic dyslipidemia: Pharmacotherapy to reduce cardiovascular risk', *Pharmacology & Therapeutics*, 2010;126:314–45

99. AIM-High Investigators, 'Niacin in patients with low HDL cholesterol levels receiving intensive statin therapy' *New England Journal of Medicine*, 2011 Dec 15;365(24):2255–67

100. M.J. Stampfer, 'Vitamin E consumption and the risk of coronary disease in women', *New England Journal of Medicine*, 1993 May;1444–9

101. E.B. Rimm, et al., 'Vitamin E consumption and the risk of coronary heart disease in men', *New England Journal of Medicine*, 1993 May;1450–5

102. K.G. Losonczy, et al. 'Vitamin E and vitamin C supplement use and risk of all- cause and coronary heart disease mortality in older persons: The Established Populations for Epidemiologic Studies of the Elderly', *American Journal of Clinical Nutrition*, 1996 Aug;64(2):190–6

103. R. Pfister, S.J. Sharp, et al., 'Plasma vitamin C predicts incident heart failure in men and women in European Prospective Investigation into Cancer and Nutrition-Norfolk prospective study', *American Heart Journal*, 2011 Aug;162(2):246–53

104. N. Stephens, et al., 'Randomised controlled trial of vitamin E in patients with coronary disease: Cambridge Heart Antioxidant Study (CHAOS)', *Lancet*, 1996 Mar;347

105. B. Manuel, Y. Keenoy, et al., 'Impact of Vitamin E supplementation on lipoprotein peroxidation and composition in Type 1 diabetic patients treated with Atorvastatin', *Atherosclerosis*, 2004 Aug;175(2):369–76

106. B. Debreceni, L. Debreceni, 'Why do homocysteine-lowering B vitamin and antioxidant E vitamin supplementations appear to be ineffective in the prevention of cardiovascular diseases?', *Cardiovascular Therapy*, 2011 Apr. [Epub ahead of print]

107. Heck, et al., 'Potential interactions between alternative therapies and warfarin', *American Journal of Health-System Pharmacy*, 2000;57: 1221–30

108. P.K. Myint, R.N. Luben, et al., 'Association between plasma vitamin C concentrations and blood pressure in the European prospective investigation into cancer-norfolk population-based study', *Hypertension*, 2011 Sep;58(3):372–9

109. O. Osilesi, et al., 'Blood pressure and plasma lipids during ascorbic acid supplementation in borderline hypertensive and normotensive adults', *Nutrition Research*, 1991;11:405–12

110. P. Jacques, 'Effects of vitamin C on high density lipoprotein cholesterol and blood pressure', *American Journal of the College of Nutrition*, 1992;11(2):139–44; see also S.J. Duffy, et al., 'Treatment of hypertension with ascorbic acid', *Lancet*, 1999;354(9195): 2048–9

111. S.P. Juraschek et al., 'Effects of vitamin C supplementation on blood pressure: a meta-analysis of randomised controlled trials', *American Journal of Clinical Nutrition* 2012 May;95(5):1079–88

112. P. Knekt, et al., 'Antioxidant vitamins and coronary heart disease risk: A pooled analysis of 9 cohorts', *American Journal of Clinical Nutrition*, 2004;80(6): 1508–20

113. S. Möhlenkamp, et al.,'Quantification of coronary atherosclerosis and inflammation to predict coronary events and all-cause mortality', *Journal of the American College of Cardiologists*, 2011 Mar 29;57(13):1455–64

114. *American Journal of Clinical Nutrition*, 1996;64:90–6

115. M. Shargorodsky, O. Debby, et al., 'Effect of long-term treatment with antioxidants (vitamin C, vitamin E, coenzyme Q10 and selenium) on arterial compliance, humoral factors and inflammatory markers in patients with multiple cardiovascular risk factors', *Nutrition Metabolism and Cardiovascular Diseases Journal*, 2010;7: 55

116. K. Jones, et al., 'Coenzyme Q-10 and cardiovascular health', *Alternative Therapies in Health Medicine*, 2004 Jan-Feb;10(1):22–30; see also M. Dhanasekaran and J. Ren, 'The emerging role of coenzyme Q-10 in aging, neurodegeneration, cardiovascular disease, cancer and diabetes mellitus', *Current Neurovascular Research*, 2005 Dec;2(5):447–59

117. K. Jones, et al., 'Coenzyme Q-10 and cardiovascular health', *Alternative Therapies in Health Medicine*, 2004 Jan-Feb;10(1):22–30; see also M. Dhanasekaran and J. Ren, 'The emerging role of coenzyme Q-10 in aging, neurodegeneration, cardiovascular disease, cancer and diabetes mellitus', *Current Neurovascular Research*, 2005 Dec;2(5):447–59

118. P. Langsjoen and A. Langsjoen, 'Overview of the use of CoQ10 in cardiovascular disease,' *Biofactors*, 1999;9(21–4):273–84

119. K. Folkers, Y. Yamamura, *Biomedical and Clinical Aspects of Coexzyme Q* (1986), Elsevier Science Publishers

120. K. Folkers, Y. Yamamura, *Biomedical and Clinical Aspects of Coexzyme Q* (1986), Elsevier Science Publishers

121. F. Rosenfeldt, et al., 'Response of the senescent heart to stress: Clinical therapeutic strategies and quest for mitochondrial predictors of biological age', *Annals of the NY Academy of Sciences*, 2004;1019:78–84 see also: F. Rosenfeldt, et al., 'CoEnzyme Q10 therapy before cardiac surgery improves mitochondrial function and in vitro contractility of myocardial tissue', *Journal of the Thoracical and Cardiovascular Surgery*, 2005;129(1):25–32

122. L. Tiano, et al., 'Effect of coenzyme Q_{10} administration on endothelial function and extracellular superoxide dismutase in patients with ischaemic heart disease: A double-blind, randomized controlled study', *European Heart Journal*, 2007;28(18):2249–55

123. R. Belardinelli, et al., 'Coenzyme Q10 improves contractility of dysfunctional myocardium in chronic heart failure', *Biofactors*, 2005; 25(1–4):137–45

124. F. Rosenfeldt, et al., 'Coenzyme Q10 therapy before cardiac surgery improves mitochondrial function and in vitro contractility of myocardial tissue', *Journal of Thoracic and Cardiovascular Surgery*, 2005 Jan;129(1):25–32

125. R.B. Singh, et al., 'Effect of coenzyme Q10 on risk of atherosclerosis in patients with recent myocardial infarction' *Molecular and Cellular Biochemistry*, 2003 Apr;246(1–2):75–82

126. P.H. Langsjoen, et al., 'Treatment of statin adverse effects with supplemental Coenzyme Q10 and statin drug discontinuation', *Biofactors*, 2005; 25(1–4):147–52

127. K. Jones, et al., 'Coenzyme Q-10 and cardiovascular health', *Alternative Therapies in Health & Medicine*, 2004;10(1):22–30; see also M. Dhanasekaran and J. Ren, 'The emerging role of coenzyme Q-10 in aging, neurodegeneration, cardiovascular disease, cancer and diabetes mellitus', *Current Neurovascular Research*, 2005;2(5):447–59

128. P.H. Langsjoen and A.M. Langsjoen 'Supplemental ubiquinol in patients with advanced congestive heart failure', *BioFactors*, 2008;32: 119–128

129. P. Jong-Gil, O. Goo Taeg, 'The role of peroxidases in the pathogenesis of atherosclerosis', *Biochemistry and Molecular Biology Reports*, 2011;44(8): 497–505

130. K.R. Gibson, T.J. Winterburn, et al., 'Therapeutic potential of N-acetylcysteine as an antiplatelet agent in patients with type-2 diabetes', *Cardiovascular Diabetology*, 2011 May;10:43.

131. National Diet and Nutritional Survey, 2009, FSA

132. K. Park, D. Mozaffarian, 'Omega-3 fatty acids, mercury, and selenium in fish and the risk of cardiovascular diseases', *Current Atherosclerosis Reports*, 2010 Nov;12(6):414–22

133. X. Wang, Y. Yu, et al., 'Alpha-lipoic acid protects against myocardial ischemia/reperfusion injury via multiple target effects', *Food and Chemical Toxicology*, 2011 Aug [Epub ahead of print]

134. L. Steffen, 'Eat your fruit and vegetables', *Lancet*, 2006;367:278–9

135. M.G. Shrime, S.R. Bauer, et al., 'Flavonoid-rich cocoa consumption affects multiple cardiovascular risk factors in a meta-analysis of short-term studies', *Journal of Nutrition*, 2011 Nov;141(11):1982–8

136. K. Lee, et al., 'Cocoa has more phenolic phytochemicals and a higher antioxidant capacity than teas and red wine', *Journal of the Agricultural and Food Chemistry*, 2003 Dec;51(25):7292–5

137. M. Serafini, et al., 'Plasma antioxidants from chocolate', *Nature*, 2003 Aug;424(6952):1013

138. P.C. Elwood, et al., 'Magnesium and calcium in the myocardium: Cause of death and area differences', *Lancet*, 1980 Oct;316(8197):720–2; see also P. Turlapaty, and B. Altura, 'Magnesium deficiency produces spasms of coronary arteries: Relationship to etiology of sudden death ischemic heart disease', *Science*, 1980 Apr;208:198–200

139. B. Altura and B. Altura, 'Magnesium in cardiovascular biology', *Scientific American*, 1995 May/June;28–36

140. S.C. Larsson, N.Orsini, A.Wolk, 'Dietary magnesium intake and risk of stroke: A meta-analysis', *American Journal of Clinical Nutrition*, 2012 [Epub ahead of print]

141. W.J. Mroczek, et al., 'Effect of magnesium sulfate on cardiovascular hemodynamics', *Angiology*, 1977;28(10):720–4

142. C.M. Champagne, 'Magnesium in hypertension, cardiovascular disease,

metabolic syndrome, and other conditions: a review', *Nutrition in Clinical Practice*, 2008 Apr-May;23(2):142–51

143. L.S. Hatzistavri, P.A. Sarafidis, et al., 'Oral magnesium supplementation reduces ambulatory blood pressure in patients with mild hypertension', *American Journal of Hypertension*, 2009 Oct;22(10):1070–5

144. B.T. Altura and B.M. Altura, 'Magnesium in cardiovascular biology', *Scientific American*, 1995 May–June;28–36

145. D. Almoznino-Sarafian, S. Berman, et al., 'Magnesium and C-reactive protein in heart failure: an anti-inflammatory effect of magnesium administration?', *European Journal of Nutrition*, 2007 Jun;46(4):230–7

146. L. Hooper, et al., 'Advice to reduce dietary salt for prevention of cardiovascular disease', *Cochrane Database of Systematic Reviews*, 2004:CD003656

147. http://news.bbc.co.uk/1/hi/health/6570933.stm

148. R.S. Taylor, et al. 'Reduced dietary salt for the prevention of cardiovascular disease: a meta-analysis of randomized controlled trials (Cochrane review)', *American Journal of Hypertension*, 2011 Aug;24:843–53

149. P. Strazzullo, et al., 'Salt intake, stroke, and cardiovascular disease: meta-analysis of prospective studies', *British Medical Journal*, 2009;339:b4567

150. M.C. Houston, K.J. Harper 'Potassium, magnesium, and calcium: Their role in both the cause and treatment of hypertension', *Journal of Clinical Hypertension (Greenwich)*, 2008 Jul;10(7 Suppl 2):3–11

151. A. Masood, et al., 'Serum high sensitivity C-reactive protein levels and the severity of coronary atherosclerosis assessed by angiographic gensini score', *Journal of the Pakistan Medical Association*, 2011 Apr;61(4):325–7

152. M. Di Napoli, et al., 'C-reactive protein level measurement improves mortality prediction when added to the spontaneous intracerebral hemorrhage score', *Stroke*, 2011 May;42(5):1230–6

153. B. Zhang B, et al., 'The relationships between erythrocyte membrane n-6 to n-3 polyunsaturated fatty acids ratio and blood lipids and C-reactive protein in Chinese adults: an observational study', *Biomedical and Environmental Sciences*, 2011 Jun;24(3):234–42

154. J. de Batlle, et al., 'Association between Ω3 and Ω6 fatty acid intakes and serum inflammatory markers in COPD', *Journal of Nutritional Biochemistry*, 2011 Sep 1 [Epub ahead of print]

155. S. Devaraj, et al., 'Gamma-tocopherol supplementation alone and in combination with alpha-tocopherol alters biomarkers of oxidative stress and inflammation in subjects with metabolic syndrome', *Free Radical Biology & Medicine*, 2008: 44:1203–8

156. M.R. Rizzo, et al., 'Evidence for anti-inflammatory effects of combined administration of vitamin E and C in older persons with impaired fasting glucose: Impact on insulin action', *Journal of the American College of Nutrition*, 2008; 27:505–11

157. R. Castillo, et al., 'Antioxidant therapy reduces oxidative and inflammatory tissue damage in patients subjected to cardiac surgery with extracorporeal

circulation', *Basic Clinical Pharmacology and Toxicology*, 2011 Apr;108(4):256–62

158. W. Wongcharoen, A. Phrommintikul, 'The protective role of curcumin in cardiovascular diseases', *International Journal of Cardiology*, 2009 Apr;133(2):145–51

159. B. Ovbiagele, 'Potential role of curcumin in stroke prevention', *Expert Review of Neurotherapeutics*, 2008Aug;8(8):1175–6

160. H. Ghanim, et al., 'An anti-inflammatory and reactive oxygen species suppressive effects of an extract of polygonum cuspidatum containing resveratrol', *The Journal of Clinical Endocrinology & Metabolism*, 95:E1–8.

161. Shakeri, et al., 'Effects of L-carnitine supplement on serum inflammatory cytokines, C-reactive protein, lipoprotein (a), and oxidative stress in hemodialysis patients with Lp (a) hyperlipoproteinemia', *Hemodialysis International*, 14:498–504

162. B. Bao, et al., 'Zinc decreases C-reactive protein, lipid peroxidation, and inflammatory cytokines in elderly subjects: a potential implication of zinc as an atheroprotective agent', *The American Journal of Clinical Nutrition*, 91:1634–41

163. E.B. Levitan, et al., 'Dietary glycemic index, dietary glycemic load, blood lipids, and C-reactive protein', *Metabolism*, 2008 Mar;57(3):437–43

164. L. Galland, 'Diet and inflammation', *Nutrition in Clinical Practractice*, 2010 Dec;25(6):634–40

165. North, et al., 'The effects of dietary fiber on C-reactive protein, an inflammation marker predicting cardiovascular disease', *European Journal of Clinical Nutrition*, 2009;63:921–33

166. L.A. Daray, et al., 'Endurance and resistance training lowers C-reactive protein in young, healthy females', *Applied Physiology, Nutrition, and Metabolism* 2011 Oct 4. [Epub ahead of print]

167. A. Prentice and S. Jebb, 'Obesity in Britain: Gluttony or sloth?', *British Medical Journal*, 1995;311:437–9

168. S. Yusuf, et al., 'Effect of potentially modifiable risk factors associated with myocardial infarction in 52 countries (the INTERHEART study): Case-control study', *Lancet*, 2004 Sep;364(9438):937–52

169. P. Kokkinos, et al., 'Exercise capacity and mortality in older men: A 20-year follow-up study', *Circulation*, 2010 Aug;122(8):790–7

170. Jane Østergaard Pedersen, et al., 'The combined influence of leisure-time physical activity and weekly alcohol intake on fatal ischaemic heart disease and all-cause mortality', *European Heart Journal*, 2008;29: 204–12

171. W. McArdle, chapter in *Medical Aspects of Clinical Nutrition* (1983), Keats Publishing

172. S. Balducci, et al., 'Effect of an intensive exercise intervention strategy on modifiable cardiovascular risk factors in subjects with type 2 diabetes mellitus: A randomized controlled trial: The Italian Diabetes and Exercise Study (IDES)', *Archives of Internal Medicine*, 2010 Nov;170(20):1794–803

173. C.J. Kim, et al., 'Effects of a cardiovascular risk reduction intervention

with psychobehavioral strategies for Korean adults with type 2 diabetes and metabolic syndrome', *Journal of Cardiovascular Nursing*, 2011 Mar–Apr;26(2):117–28

174. W.J. Kraemer, et al., 'Effects of heavy-resistance training on hormonal response patterns in younger vs. older men', *Journal of Applied Physiology*, 1999 Sep;87(3):982–92

175. M.K. Malinski, et al., 'Alcohol consumption and cardiovascular disease mortality in hypertensive men', *Archives of Internal Medicine* 2004; 164:623–8

176. Review on alcohol and cardiovascular disease risk – see http://pubs.niaaa.nih.gov/publications/arh25-4/255-261.htm

177. L. Wang, et al., 'Alcohol consumption, weight gain, and risk of becoming overweight in middle-aged and older women', *Archives of Internal Medicine*, 2010 Mar ;170(5):453–61

178. W. Nseir, et al., 'Soft drinks consumption and nonalcoholic fatty liver disease', *World Journal of Gastroenterology*, 2010 Jun;16(21):2579–88

179. H.K. Choi and G. Curhan, 'Soft drinks, fructose consumption, and the risk of gout in men: Prospective cohort study', *British Medical Journal*, 2008 Feb 9;336(7639):309–12

180. R. Urgert, et al., ' Comparison of effect of cafetière and filtered coffee on serum concentrations of liver aminotransferases and lipids: Six month randomised controlled trial', *British Medical Journal*, 1996 Nov;313(7069):1362–6

181. A. D'Amicis, et al., ' Italian style brewed coffee: Effect on serum cholesterol in young men', *International Journal of Epidemiology*, 1996 Jun;25(3): 513–20

Part 3

1. K.B. Scribner, et al., 'Hepatic steatosis and increased adiposity in mice consuming rapidly vs. slowly absorbed carbohydrate', *Obesity (Silver Spring)*, 2007 Sep;15(9):2190–9

2. D. Thomas, et al., *The Cochrane Library*, 2007

3. G. Yang, et al., 'Longitudinal study of soy food intake and blood pressure among middle-aged and elderly Chinese women', *American Journal of Clinical Nutrition*, 2005;81(5),1012–1017

4. M. Yoshida, et al., 'Effect of plant sterols and glucomannan on lipids in individuals with and without type II diabetes', *European Journal of Clinical Nutrition*, 2006 Apr;60(4):529–3; also H. L. Chen, et al., 'Konjac supplement alleviated hypercholesterolemia and hyperglycemia in type-2 diabetic subjects: A randomized double-blind trial', *Journal of the American College of Nutrition*, 2003 Feb;22(1):36–42

5. A. Lewis, et al., 'Treatment of hypertriglyceridemia with omega-3 fatty acids: A systemic review', *Journal of the American Academy of Nurse Practitioners*, 2004 Sep;16(9):384–5

6.   M.D. Ashen and R.S. Blumenthal, 'Low HDL Cholesterol Levels', *New England Journal of Medicine*, 2005 Sep;353;1252–60
7.   I. Singh, et al., 'High-density lipoprotein as a therapeutic target a systematic review', *Journal of the American Medical Association*, 2007 Aug;298:7
8.   See http://www.nlm.nih.gov/medlineplus/druginfo/natural/patient-niacin. html
9.   S.M. Grundy, et al., 'Efficacy, safety, and tolerability of once-daily niacin for the treatment of dyslipidemia associated with type 2 diabetes: Results of the assessment of diabetes control and evaluation of the efficacy of niaspan trial', *Archives of Internal Medicine*, 2002 Jul;162(14):1568–76
10.   W.J. Mroczek, et al., 'Effect of magnesium sulfate on cardiovascular hemodynamics', *Angiology* 1977;28, 720–4
11.   B.T. Altura and B.M. Altura, 'Magnesium in cardiovascular biology', *Scientific American*, 1995;28–36
12.   K. Dunder, 'Increase in blood glucose concentration during antihypertensive treatment as a predictor of myocardial infarction: Population based cohort study', *British Medical Journal*, 2003 Mar;326:681
13.   B.R. Davis, et al., 'Role of diuretics in the prevention of heart failure: The Antihypertensive and Lipid-Lowering Treatment to Prevent Heart Attack Trial', *Circulation*, 2006 May;113(18):2201–10
14.   S. Vasdev, et al., 'Prevention of fructose-induced hypertension by dietary vitamins', *Clinical Biochemistry*, 2004 Jan;37:1–9
15.   M.W. Brands, et al., 'Obesity and hypertension: Roles of hyperinsulinemia, sympathetic nervous system and intrarenal mechanisms', *Journal of Nutrition*, Supplement 1995 Jun;125(6): 1725–1731
16.   P. Holford, et al., 'The effects of a low glycemic load diet on weight loss and key health risk indicators', *Journal of Orthomolecular Medicine*, 2006;21(2)
17.   M. Houston and K. Harper, 'Potassium, magnesium, and calcium: Their role in both the cause and treatment of hypertension', *Journal of Clincal Hypertension*, 2008 July;10(7):3–11
18.   K.E. Charlton, et al., 'A food-based dietary strategy lowers blood pressure in a low socio-economic setting: A randomised study in South Africa', *Public Health Nutrition*, 2008 Dec;11(12):1397–406
19.   J. Geleijnse, et al., 'Reduction of blood pressure with a low sodium, high potassium, high magnesium salt in older subjects with mild to moderate hypertension', *British Medical Journal*, 1994;309:436–40
20.   A.J. Webb, et al., 'Acute blood pressure lowering, vasoprotective, and antiplatelet properties of dietary nitrate via bioconversion to nitrite', *Hypertension*, 2008 Mar;51:784–790
21.   T.A. Mori, 'Omega-3 fatty acids and hypertension in humans', *Clinical and Experimental Pharmacology and Physiology*, 2006 Sep;33(9):842–6
22.   R. Rodrigo, et al., 'Relationship between oxidative stress and essential hypertension', *Hypertension Research*, 2007;30(12):1159–67
23.   S. Zibadi, 'Reduction of cardiovascular risk factors in subjects with type 2 diabetes by Pycnogenol supplementation', *Nutrition Research*, 2008;28:315–20

24. W.V. Judy, J.H. Hall, et al., 'Double blind-double crossover study of coenzyme Q10 in heart failure', in K. Folkers, Y. Yamamura, *Biomedical and Clinical Aspects of Coexzyme Q* (1986), Elsevier Science Publishers: 315–23

25. B. Burke, 'Randomized, double blind, placebo-controlled trial of CoQ_{10} in isolated systolic hypertension', *Southern Medical Journal*, 2001;94(11):1112–7

26. J.M. Hodgson, et al., 'Coenzyme Q10 improves blood pressure and glycemic control: a controlled trial in subjects with type 2 diabetes', *European Journal of Clinical Nutrition*, 2002;56(11):1137–1142

27. D.A. McCarron, 'Calcium metabolism in hypertension', *Keio Journal of Medicine*, 1995;44(4):105–14

28. A. Poduri, et al., 'Effect of ACE inhibitors and beta-blockers on homocysteine levels in essential hypertension', *Journal of Human Hypertension*, 2008 Apr;22(4):289–94

29. Reported at the American Society of Hypertension 2008 Annual Meeting

30. D. Taubert, et al., 'Effects of low habitual cocoa intake on blood pressure and bioactive nitric oxide a randomized controlled trial', *Journal of the American Medicine Association*, 2007;298(1):49–60

31. R.N. Iyer, A.A. Khan, et al., 'L-carnitine moderately improves the exercise tolerance in chronic stable angina', *Journal of the Association of Physicians of India*, 2000 Nov;48(11):1050–2

32. C.J. McMackin, M.E. Widlansky, et al., 'Effect of combined treatment with alpha-lipoic acid and acetyl-L-carnitine on vascular function and blood pressure in patients with coronary artery disease', *Journal of Clinical Hypertension (Greenwich)*, 2007 Apr;9(4):249–55

33. R. Ferrari, E. Merli, et al., 'Therapeutic effects of l-carnitine and propionyl-l-carnitine on cardiovascular diseases: A review'. Annals New York Academy of Science. 2004 Nov;1033:79–91

34. L.T. Chappell and J.P. Stahl, 'The correlation between EDTA chelation therapy and improvement in cardiovascular function: A meta-analysis', *Journal of Advancement in Medicine*, 1993;6(3)

35. C. Hancke and K. Flytlie, 'Benefit of EDTA chelation therapy in arteriosclerosis: A retrospective study of 470 patients', *Journal of Advancement in Medicine* 1993;6(3)161–171

36. C.J. Rudolph, E.W. McDonagh, et al., 'A nonsurgical approach to obstructive carotid stenosis using EDTA chelation', *Journal of Advancement in Medicine* 1991;4(3)157–166.

37. L.T. Chappell, R. Shukla, et al., 'Subsequent cardiac and stroke events in patients with known vascular disease treated with EDTA chelation therapy', *Evidence Based Integrative Medicine*, 2005;2:27–35

38. T. Jeerakathil, et al., 'Short-term risk for stroke is doubled in persons with newly treated type 2 diabetes compared with persons without diabetes', *Stroke*, 2007;38:1739

39. H. Iso, et al., 'Intake of fish and omega-3 fatty acids and risk of stroke in women', *Journal of the American Medical Association*, 2001 Jan;285(3): 304–12

40. H.J. Cho and Y.J. Kim, 'Efficacy and safety of oral citicoline in acute ischemic stroke: Drug surveillance study in 4,191 cases', *Methods & Findings in Experimental and Clinical Pharmacology*, 2009 Apr;31(3): 171–6

41. W.M. Clark, et al., 'A randomized efficacy trial of citicoline in patients with acute ischemic stroke', *Stroke*, 1999 Dec;30(12): 2592–7
see also: W.M. Clark, et al., 'A phase III randomized efficacy trial of 2000 mg citicoline in acute ischemic stroke patients', *Neurology*, 2001 Nov;57(9):1595–1602

42. J, Alvarez-Sabín and G.C. Román, 'Citicoline in vascular cognitive impairment and vascular dementia after stroke', *Stroke*, 2011 Jan;42(1):S40–3

43. A. Cherubini, et al., 'Antioxidant Profile and Early Outcome in Stroke Patients', *Stroke*, 2000;31:2295

44. Y. Wang, et al., 'Dietary supplementation with blueberries, spinach, or spirulina reduces ischemic brain damage', *Experimental Neurology*, 2005 May;193(1):75–84

45. J. Hee Kang, et al., 'Vitamin E, vitamin C, beta carotene, and cognitive function among women with or at risk of cardiovascular disease: The Women's Antioxidant and Cardiovascular Study', *Circulation*, 2009 Jun 2;119(21):2772–80

46. P.K. Myint, et al., 'Plasma vitamin C concentrations predict risk of incident stroke over 10 y in 20.649 participants of the European Prospective Investigation into Cancer–Norfolk prospective population study', *American Journal of Clinical Nutrition*, 2008 Jan;87(1): 64–9

47. M. Schürks, et al., 'Effects of vitamin E on stroke subtypes: Meta-analysis of randomized controlled trials', *British Medical Journal*, 2010;341:c5702

48. G.L. Lenzi, et al., 'Post-stroke depression', *Revue Neurologique*, 2008 Oct;164 (10):837–40

49. Wang, et al., 'Efficacy of folic acid supplementation in stroke prevention: a meta-analysis', *Lancet*, 2007 Jun;369(9576):1876–1882

50. E.P. Quinlivan, et al., 'Importance of both folic acid and vitamin B_{12} in reduction of risk of vascular disease', *Lancet*, 2002 Jan;359:227–8

Part 4

1. J. Warren, et al., 'Low glycemic index breakfasts and reduced food intake in preadolescent children', *Pediatrics*, 2003;112(5):414

2. D. Ludwig, 'Dietary glycemic index and regulation of body weight', *Lipids*, 2003;38(2):117–21

3. K. Heaton, et al., 'Particle size of wheat, maize and oat test meals: Effects on plasma glucose and insulin responses and on the rate of starch digestion in vitro', *American Journal of Clinical Nutrition*, 1988;47:675–82

4. E. Cheraskin, 'The breakfast/lunch/dinner ritual', *Journal of Orthomolecular Medicine*, 1993;8(1):6–10

5.   J. T. Braaten, et al., 'High beta-glucan oat bran and oat gum reduce postprandial blood glucose and insulin in subjects with and without type 2 diabetes', *Diabetic Medicine*, 1994;11(3):312–18

6.   J. Uribarri, et al., 'Advanced glycation end products in foods and a practical guide to their reduction in the diet', *Journal of the American Dietetic Association*, 2010 Jun;110(6):911–16

7.   S. Rautiainen, et al., 'Multivitamin use and the risk of myocardial infarction: A population-based cohort of Swedish women', *American Journal of Clinical Nutrition*, 2010 Nov;92(5):1251–6

8.   Jonathan Myers, PhD 'Exercise and cardiovascular health', *Circulation*, 2003;107:e2–e5

9.   P. Thompson, et al., 'Exercise and physical activity in the prevention and treatment of atherosclerotic cardiovascular disease: A statement from the Council on Clinical Cardiology', *Circulation*, 2003;107:3109–16

10. P. Holford, et al., *100% Health Survey* (2010), Holford and Associates

11. A. Peters, 'The selfish brain: Competition for energy resources', *American Journal of Human Biology*, 2010 Nov [Epub ahead of print]

12. P. Holford, et al., 'The effects of a low glycemic load diet on weight loss and key health risk indicators', *Journal of Orthomolecular Medicine*, 2006;21(2):71–8

13. N. Ranjit, et al., 'Psychosocial factors and inflammation in the multi-ethnic study of atherosclerosis', *Archives of Internal Medicine*, 2007;167:174–81

14. R. McCraty and D. Tomasino, 'Emotional stress, positive emotions and psychophysiological coherence', in *Stress in Health and Disease* (2006), Wiley:342–65

Recommended Reading

The Great Cholesterol Con, Dr Malcolm Kendrick, John Blake (2008)

The Cholesterol Myths, Dr Uffe Ravnskov, New Trends Publishing (2000)

How to Quit Without Feeling S**t, Patrick Holford, David Miller and James Braly, Little, Brown Book Group (2008)

Transforming Stress, Deborah Rozman and Doc Lew Childre, New Harbinger Publications (2005)

Take the Pressure off Your Heart, Robert Kowalski, Struik Publishers (2006)

The Low-GL Diet Cookbook, Patrick Holford and Fiona McDonald Joyce, Piatkus (2005)

The 10 Secrets of 100% Health Cookbook, Patrick Holford and Fiona McDonald Joyce, Piatkus (2012)

Ready, Set, Go!, Phil Campbell, Pristine Publishers (2002)

Say No to Diabetes, Patrick Holford, Piatkus (2011)

Resources

Nutritional therapy and consultations To find a recommended nutritional therapist near you, visit the British Association for Applied Nutrition and Nutritional Therapy at www.bant.org.uk. This website provides details of who to see both in the UK and internationally. If you are unable to find any practitioners in your area, you can always take an online assessment (see below).

Online 100% Health Programme Are you 100% healthy? Find out with a health check and comprehensive 100% Health Programme, which will give you a personalised action plan, including diet and supplements. Visit www.patrickholford.com.

Chelation therapy is available, in the UK, from these medical doctors:

Dr L. Zieger, 56 Knockomie Rise, Forres IV36 2HG, Scotland, tel.: 01309 673100

Dr P. Idahosa, Institute of Natural Medicine and Preventive Cardiology, 128 Winchester Road, London N9 9EE, tel.: 07956 224299

Dr Rodney Adeniyi-Jones, Genesis Wellness, 50 New Cavendish Street, London W1G 8TL, tel: 0207 486 6358

HeartMath The HeartMath stress-relieving EM-Wave Monitor is available from www.patrickholford.com. In the UK you can attend workshops called Transforming Stress into Resilience, to hardwire these simple stress-busting techniques, or you can also consult a practitioner on a one-to-one basis. See www.patrickholford.com/heartmath for more details on these products and workshops.

Psychocalisthenics is an excellent exercise system that takes less than 20 minutes a day, and develops strength, suppleness and stamina as well as generating vital energy. The best way to learn it is to do the Psychocalisthenics Training. See www.patrickholford.com (events) for details. Also available are the book *Master Level Exercise: Psychocalisthenics* and the Psychocalisthenics CD and DVD, available from www.patrickholford.com (shop). For further information please see www.pcals.com.

Resistance training exercises Visit www.holforddiet.com for information on fat-burning exercises (see the right-hand side of the home page) that can be easily included in your exercise plan. Also, to see the video of Dr Joseph Mercola's Peak 8 system, visit:

http://fitness.mercola.com/sites/fitness/archive/2010/11/13/phil-campbell-on-peak-8-exercises.aspxor find out more at his website www.readysteadygofitness.com.

Zest4Life is a health and nutrition club, based on low-GL principles, that provides advice, coaching and support for losing weight and gaining health through a series of weekly meetings. For more information, visit www.zest4life.com. Also see page 153 for more details.

Laboratory tests

Homocysteine and GL Check (measures your level of glycosylated haemoglobin, also called HbA1C) tests are available through YorkTest Laboratories, using a home-test kit where you can take your own pinprick blood sample and return it to the lab for analysis. Visit www.yorktest.com, or call freephone (UK) 0800 074 6185. These test kits are also available from www.totallynourish.com and www. healthproductsforlife.com.

Other tests

You may also want to measure your **C-reactive protein (hs CRP)** or complete an in-depth assessment of your CV Health measuring a spectrum of key measures such as HDL cholesterol, LDL cholesterol, triglycerides, lipoprotein(a), homocysteine, hs-CRP, vitamin D and fibrinogen in one test. Speak to your nutritional therapist, health-care professional or doctor, who can arrange these tests.

Health products

Cherry Active is sold in a highly concentrated juice format. Mix a 30ml serving of the concentrate with 250ml water to make a deliciously healthy, low-GL cherry juice with a high ORAC score. Each 946ml bottle contains the juice from over 3,000 cherries – that's half a tree's worth – and contains a month's supply. Cherry Active is also available as a dried cherry snack and in capsules. For more information and to order, visit www.totallynourish.com (see below).

Chia seeds, the highest vegetarian source of omega-3, are available from www.totallynourish.com. If you'd like to find out more, two useful websites are www.eatchia.com and www.drcoateschia.com.

Essential Balance by Higher Nature and Udo's Choice are two good seed oil blends that are available in health-food stores.

Get Up & Go, my low-GL breakfast shake powder, is available in most health-food stores or by mail order. Visit www.totallynourish. com.

Glucomannan, and **konjac fibre** are available from most health-food stores or by mail order. Visit www.totallynourish.com. **PGX** is currently not available in the UK. For more details and a supplier abroad, visit www.pgx.com.

Sugar alternative – xylitol is a low-GL natural sugar alternative – available in many supermarkets and health-food stores under various names such as XyloBrit and Total Sweet. Available online from www. totallynourish.com.

Supplements

Finding your own perfect supplement programme can be confusing, but my website, www.patrickholford.com, offers useful guidance. In this section are examples of supplements that provide the nutrients at the levels discussed in this book. The addresses of the companies whose products I've referred to are given at the end.

Multivitamin and mineral supplements

Supplementing the right multivitamin is the most important supplement decision you make. Most multis are based on RDA levels of nutrients, which are not the same as optimum nutrition levels. A good multivitamin based on optimum nutrition levels is Holford's Advanced Optimum Nutrition Formula. Another is Solgar's Formula VM2000. Both of these recommend taking two tablets a day. Advanced Optimum Nutrition Formula has higher mineral levels, especially for calcium and magnesium.

Essential fats and fish oil supplements

The most important omega-3 fats are DHA, DPA and EPA, found both in oily fish and in cod liver oil. The most important omega-6 fat is GLA, the richest source being borage (also known as starflower) oil. In all you are looking for at least 600mg of combined EPA, DPA and DHA a day.

Try BioCare's Mega-EPA, a high-potency omega-3 fish oil supplement. They also produce Essential Omegas, which provides a highly concentrated mix of EPA, DHA, DPA and GLA. Seven Seas produce Extra High Strength Cod Liver Oil.

Vitamin C

Vitamin C is available in tablets and powders. Look for one which contains synergistic antioxidant nutrients such as zinc, black elderberry extracts and anthocyanidins. Complexes of vitamin C with bioflavonoids are available from the Holford and Solgar ranges. Biocare's Magnesium Ascorbate powder provides both vitamin C and magnesium combined.

Antioxidant complex

A good all-round antioxidant complex should provide glutathione or N-acetyl-cysteine (NAC), alpha-lipoic acid, vitamin E, vitamin C (not so essential as it is included in the basics), CoQ_{10}, resveratrol, anthocyanidins of berry extracts, zinc, selenium, carotenoids and vitamin A. Two products that fulfil these criteria are Holford's AGE Antioxidant and Solgar's Advanced Antioxidant Nutrients. You can also get supplements of just alpha-lipoic acid or CoQ_{10}. Holford's CoQ_{10} + Carnitine provides a combination of the amino acid carnitine and CoQ_{10}. Two capsules provide 400mg of carnitine plus 60mg of CoQ_{10}.

Sugar balance and weight maintenance

Look for a product that contains 200mcg of chromium, either as chromium polynicotinate or as chromium picolinate, ideally with a cinnamon high in MCHP (Cinnulin PF® is the name of a concentrated extract of cinnamon that is especially high in MCHP). Try Cinnachrome, which combines chromium, cinnamon extract and niacin. Chromium may also be supplied with either garcinia cambogia (high in HCA) or 5-HTP, which are primarily included to help weight loss. GL Support combines these with B vitamins. Holford's CarboSlow provides glucomannan fibre. In the US and Canada another superfibre that lowers the GL of a meal is PGX, widely available in health-food stores and online.

High-dose niacin

The non-blushing form of niacin is called inositol hexanicotinate. Solgar have a 500mg Non-Flush Niacin and a straight Niacin 500mg, which causes blushing. The Holford No Blush Niacin provides 500mg per capsule, together with magnesium and vitamin C. Two a day provides an additional 290mg of magnesium and 490mg of vitamin C. Slow-release niacin is also available on prescription as Niaspan.

Optional extras

Other supplements that you might want to try include homocysteine-lowering B vitamins (containing at least B_{12} 500mcg, folic acid 500mcg and B_6 20mg, magnesium, lysine, L-arginine and L-citrulline). These are available from the companies listed below.

Supplement suppliers

The following companies produce good-quality supplements that are widely available in the UK.

BioCare produce an extensive range of nutritional and herbal supplements. Their products are stocked by most good health-food stores. Visit www.biocare.co.uk, tel.: 0121 433 3727.

Patrick Holford products, including daily 'packs', are stocked in good health food stores and in Holland and Barrett stores nationwide (visit www.hollandandbarrett.com or call 0870 606 6605). They are also available by mail order from Totally Nourish – see below.

Totally Nourish is an online health shop that stocks many high-quality health products, including home test kits and supplements. Visit www.totallynourish.com, tel.: 0800 085 7749 (freephone within the UK).

Solgar Available in most independent health-food stores or visit www.solgar-vitamins.co.uk, tel.: 01442 890355.

In other regions

South Africa

The original Patrick Holford vitamin and supplement brand from the UK is now available in South Africa through leading health-food stores, Dis-Chem and Clicks retail pharmacies. For more information on availability of the range email info@holforddirect.co.za or contact 011 666 8994.

Australia

Solgar supplements are available in Australia. Visit www.solgar.com.au, tel.: 1800 029 871 (free call) for your nearest supplier. Another good brand is Blackmores.

New Zealand

BioCare and Holford products (see above) are available in New Zealand through Pacific Health. Visit www.pachealth.co.nz, tel.: 0064 9815 0707.

Singapore

BioCare, Holford (see above) and Solgar products are available in Singapore through Essential Living. Visit www.essliv.com, tel.: 6276 1380.

UAE

BioCare and Holford supplements are available in Dubai and the UAE from Organic Foods & Café, PO Box 117629, Dubai, United Arab Emirates; visit www.organicfoodsandcafe.com; tel.: +971 44340577.

Index

(page numbers in italic type indicate illustrations)